Qualitative Research in Midwifery and Childbirth

Qualitative research, particularly phenomenology, is increasingly popular as a method for midwifery and health-related research. These approaches enable rich and detailed explanations to be uncovered and bring experience to life. Important recommendations and practice-based implications may then be raised and debated for future use. This book brings together a range of phenomenological methods and insights into one accessible text.

Illustrated with plenty of examples of successful phenomenological research, *Qualitative Research in Midwifery and Childbirth* keeps the focus applied to midwifery and childbirth and makes clear the links to practice throughout. The book introduces three key phenomenological approaches – descriptive, interpretive and the life world – and includes a comparative chapter which discusses the differences between these varied perspectives and methods. Each chapter focuses on how these approaches are used within midwifery research. The remaining chapters present a number of different research projects. These demonstrate how different phenomenological approaches have been used to explore and uncover experiences of childbirth and maternity as well as offering important insights into how women experience different facets of the birth experience during the antenatal, intra-partum and postnatal period.

Designed for researchers and students undertaking research projects on midwifery and childbirth, this text includes contributions from a range of international and highly regarded phenomenological authors and researchers.

Gill Thomson is a social scientist with extensive experience of quantitative and qualitative data collection and analysis in health and social care settings. She is currently Research Fellow at the University of Central Lancashire, UK.

Fiona Dykes is Professor of Maternal and Infant Health and Director of the Maternal and Infant Nutrition and Nurture Unit (MAINN) at the University of Central Lancashire, UK. She is also an Adjunct Professor at University of Western Sydney. Fiona's research and teaching focuses on the global, socio-cultural and political influences upon infant and young child feeding practices.

Soo Downe is Professor of Midwifery Studies at the University of Central Lancashire, UK. Her main research focus is the nature of, and culture around, normal birth. She is the editor of *Normal Childbirth: Evidence and Debate* (2004, 2008), and the founder of the International Normal Birth Research conference series.

Qualitative Research in Midwifery and Childbirth

Phenomenological approaches

Edited by Gill Thomson, Fiona Dykes and Soo Downe

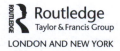

Routledge
Taylor & Francis Group

LONDON AND NEW YORK

First published 2011
by Routledge
2 Park Square, Milton Park, Abingdon, Oxon OX14 4RN

Simultaneously published in the USA and Canada
by Routledge
711 Third Avenue, New York, NY 10017

Routledge is an imprint of the Taylor & Francis Group, an informa business

British Library Cataloguing in Publication Data
A catalogue record for this book is available from the British Library

Library of Congress Cataloging in Publication Data
Qualitative research in midwifery and childbirth phenomenological
approaches / edited by Gill Thomson, Fiona Dykes, and Soo Downe. – First
edition.
p. ; cm.
Includes bibliographical references and index.
1. Midwifery–Research–Methodology. 2. Qualitative research. I. Thomson,
Gill, editor. II. Dykes, Fiona, editor. III. Downe, Soo, editor.
[DNLM: 1. Parturition. 2. Midwifery. 3. Philosophy. 4. Postnatal Care. 5.
Postpartum Period–psychology. 6. Qualitative Research. WQ 300]
RG950.Q35 2011
618.2–dc22
2010049023

ISBN: 978-0-415-57501- 0 (hbk)
ISBN: 978-0-415-57502 - 7 (pbk)
ISBN: 978-0-203-81682 - 0 (ebk)

Typeset in Baskerville
by GreenGate Publishing Services, Tonbridge, Kent

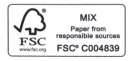

Printed and bound in Great Britain by
CPI Antony Rowe, Chippenham, Wiltshire

Contents

10 A poetic hermeneutic phenomenological analysis of midwives 'being with woman' during childbirth   172

LAUREN P. HUNTER

11 Revealing the subtle differences among postpartum mood and anxiety disorders: phenomenology holds the key   193

CHERYL TATANO BECK

12 Heidegger's contribution to hermeneutic phenomenological research   215

MARIA HEALY

13 Authenticity and poetics: what is different about phenomenology?

GILL THOMSON, FIONA DYKES AND SOO DOWNE

Contributors

Marie Berg, PhD, MNSc, PMH, RN, RM, is Professor in Health and Care Sciences with a particular focus on reproductive and perinatal health at the Institute of Health and Care Sciences, the Sahlgrenska Academy at University of Gothenburg, Sweden. She is head of the midwifery programme and master modules in Midwifery science and is also teaching in research modules. Her main current international projects are 1) the BFiN-network for developing qualitative research in childbearing in Nordic and other European countries; 2) COST action for creating a dynamic EU framework for optimal maternity care; and 3) developing nursing and midwifery education at University level in the Kivu-province, Dem. Rep. Congo. Her research aims at developing person-centred care supporting well-being in mothers and their spouses/families in the childbearing period; i.e. pregnancy, childbirth and infancy. Central theoretical standpoints for her research are the lifeworld theory and salutogenesis and she has mainly used phenomenological and hermeneutic methodologies in qualitative researches. The research is encompassed in two programmes of work: 1) Motherhood and diabetes (MODIAB) with special focus on balancing type 1 diabetes with the challenges during pregnancy, childbirth and breastfeeding period; 2) Intrapartum care, including the management of the different phases and theory development of intrapartum midwifery care to mothers and fathers/partners.

Marie is also co-editor and author of a Swedish textbook, *Support and Strengthen: Caring in Childbearing.*

Terese Bondas, PhD, Licentiate of Health Sciences, Master of Health Sciences, RN, is Professor of Nursing Science at the University of Nordland, Faculty of Professional Studies, Norway and Adjunct Professor (Methods of Health Research), Kuopio University, Faculty of Social Sciences, Finland. Terese has initialized and leads the interdisciplinary research network 'Childbearing in the European countries – a qualitative research network' (www.uin.no/bfin) that now connects 80 researchers and doctoral students (Nordforsk network 2006–2009). Research training courses and workshops in childbearing research have been organized by the network Nordic steering group attracting researchers and doctoral students from several European countries, and research collaboration has been initiated. Terese has also started and leads an interdisciplinary research network in health care leadership, NiV (www.hibo.no/niv) that unites 60 Nordic researchers, doctoral students and master level health care leaders. The steering group from Denmark, Finland, Norway and Sweden arranges research and development conferences. Terese is a member of the Caring Science Postdoctoral Research Network based at Åbo Akademi University, Finland. She has an interest to apply phenomenological and other qualitative approaches such as meta-synthesis, action research and analytic induction in her caring science research, and develop their contribution to disciplinary and evidence based care knowledge. Terese is involved in research that develops the Caritative Leadership theory that she has created, and she collaborates in several Nordic research projects in childbearing.

Joyce Cowan, MHSc (Hons) RM, RN, is currently employed as a Senior Lecturer at Auckland University of Technology in New Zealand. She is involved in undergraduate and postgraduate education and manages a small midwifery caseload providing continuity of care in the New Zealand partnership model. Since 1995 Joyce has been Director of New Zealand Action on Preeclampsia, a national charity she co-founded to raise awareness of preeclampsia, support women and families affected by the condition and raise money for research. In her capacity as Director of NZAPEC, Joyce publishes newsletters featuring women's stories of preeclampsia and reviews of current preeclampsia research. She is a regular guest lecturer at preeclampsia study days for midwives and facilitates annual updates on preeclampsia and fetal growth restriction for midwives and doctors throughout New Zealand. Joyce is a midwifery mentor and is actively involved in professional quality assurance processes within the midwifery profession.

Karin Dahlberg, PhD, ED, RN, is Professor in Caring Science, and at present Guest Professor at Linnaeus University, School of Health and Caring Sciences, Centre for Lifeworld Research, Sweden. Karin has a particular interest in continental philosophy and phenomenology, and how these ideas can strengthen the knowledge base of health care. The research has been the focus of several publications, theoretical as well as empirically derived descriptions. For many years she has given lectures on phenomenological research, in Europe as well as in the US and Asia. With the publication of the new theory of health and caring her lecture base has widened. She is also asked to serve as an expert to the national Board of Higher Education in Sweden.

Maura Dowling, PhD, MSc, BNS, RNT, RGN, RM, Cert. Oncology Nursing, is a Lecturer at the School of Nursing and Midwifery, National University of Ireland, Galway (NUI Galway). She is also programme director for the Postgraduate Diploma in Nursing (Oncology) and Master of Health

Sciences (Advanced Practice Nursing/Midwifery) at NUI Galway. Maura has extensive educational experience with midwives and nurses at postgraduate level. She has a particular interest in qualitative methodologies and has published a number of discussion papers on this topic. She has also published a number of phenomenological research studies. Maura's research interests include advanced nursing and midwifery practice. She is currently involved in a project evaluating clinical nurse and midwife specialists and advanced nurse and midwife practitioners in Ireland. She is also leading a project to help midwife and nurse specialists develop their clinical research skills and write for publication.

Soo Downe, PhD, MSc, RM, BA (Hons), spent 15 years working as a midwife in various clinical, research, and project development roles at Derby City General Hospital. In 2001 she joined the University of Central Lancashire (UCLan) in England, where she is now the Professor of Midwifery Studies. She set up the UCLan Midwifery Studies Research Unit in October 2002. She now leads the Research in Childbirth and Health (ReaCH) group. She currently chairs the UK Royal College of Midwives Campaign for Normal Birth steering committee, and she co-chairs the ICM Research Standing Committee. She has been a member of a number of national midwifery committees, and she recently chaired the joint Royal College of Obstetricians and Gynaecologists/National Patient Safety Agency subcommittee on the nature of evidence for maternity care. She was a member of the UK Medical Research Council College of Experts until it was disbanded in 2009, and she has held a number of visiting professorships, most recently in Belgium, Hong Kong, Sweden, and Australia. Her main research focus is the nature of, and culture around, normal birth. She is the editor of Normal Birth, Evidence and Debate (2004, 2008), and the founder of the International Normal Birth Research conference series.

Mel Duffy, PhD, MA, BA, is a Sociology Lecturer in the School of Nursing, Dublin City University. Mel has particular interest in lesbian health and health care, feminist theory, hermeneutical phenomenology, queer theory, identity formation, gender, sexuality and inequalities within health and society. Mel is co-founder of the first Irish MA in Sexuality Studies and the first Irish Sexuality International conference. Mel is currently collaborating on a Health Service Executive and Marte Meo project. Mel held an Irish Research Council for the Humanities and Social Sciences Postgraduate Scholarship in 2006–2007 and a Dublin City University Albert College Junior Fellowship in 2001–2002. Mel was a member of the steering group for the 2001 Health Research Board grant for the 'Empowerment of Nurses' project.

Fiona Dykes, PhD, MA, RM, ADM, Cert Ed, is Professor of Maternal and Infant Health and Director of the Maternal and Infant Nutrition and Nurture Unit (MAINN), School of Health, University of Central

Lancashire. She is also Adjunct Professor at University of Western Sydney. Fiona has a particular interest in the global, socio-cultural and political influences upon infant and young child feeding practices; she has undertaken interpretive phenomenological research with breastfeeding women in England. She has worked on WHO, UNICEF, European Union (EU Framework 6), Government (DH), NHS, UK National Institute for Health and Clinical Excellence (NICE), TrusTECH® Service Innovation (UK), British Council and Australian Research Council (ARC) funded projects. She is currently involved in projects in Africa, Australia, Sweden and Pakistan. Fiona is author of *Breastfeeding in Hospital: Mothers, Midwives and the Production Line* and co-editor (with Victoria Hall Moran) of *Maternal and Infant Nutrition and Nurture: Controversies and Challenges* and *Infant and Young Child Feeding: Challenges to implementing a Global Strategy*.

Maria Healy, RNT, MSc, PGDip RM, RGN, has been a Lecturer at the School of Nursing, Midwifery and Health Systems, University College Dublin, Ireland since January 2000. She is involved in undergraduate and postgraduate midwifery education, clinical midwifery research and engages regularly in clinical midwifery practice. Maria is currently completing her doctoral studies with the School of Health at the University of Central Lancashire. Her expertise in Heideggerian hermeneutic phenomenology originated after being awarded a scholarship from the George Mason University, Virginia and from the Iolanthe Midwifery Trust, London to attend an Institute on Heideggerian Hermeneutical Methodologies and an Institute on Interpretive Phenomenology at the George Mason University, Fairfax, Virginia, USA in June 2006.

Lauren P. Hunter, PhD, CNM, WHNP, FACNM, is Nurse-Midwife Program Director and Professor in the School of Nursing at San Diego State University, San Diego, California. She is also Adjunct Clinical Professor in the Department of Reproductive Medicine at the University of California, San Diego. She has been involved in nurse-midwifery education and clinical practice since 1987. Lauren's research trajectory emphasizes qualitative study, particularly hermeneutical phenomenology. Her research interests include the midwifery care concept of 'being with woman' during childbirth and midwifery ways of knowing. Because of her love for narrative, art, poetry and storytelling, Lauren has incorporated these aesthetic concepts into her teaching paradigm. She has published numerous articles in refereed journals that have enhanced nurse-midwifery knowledge, clinical practice, and theory. An advocate for maternal-newborn health and midwifery, Lauren has served the American College of Nurse-Midwives, locally and nationally, earning her fellowship in the college in 2006.

Marion Hunter, MA (Hons), BA, ADN, RM, RGON, is a Senior Lecturer at the School of Midwifery, Auckland University of Technology, New Zealand. For the past six years, Marion has maintained a small caseload working as a Lead Maternity Carer midwife within a rural area of New Zealand. Marion has published articles and book chapters related to birthplace and midwifery care. She has a keen interest in midwifery prescribing and is a Director of the New Zealand PHARMAC Seminar Series organizing multi-disciplinary seminars. Marion has been an Expert Advisor appointed by the New Zealand College of Midwives. In August 2010, Marion was appointed to the Midwifery Council of New Zealand (regulation authority) by the Minister of Health.

Ingela Lundgren, PhD, RM, RN, is Associate Professor at Sahlgrenska Academy, Institute of Health and Care Sciences, University of Gothenburg, Sweden and Head of Section at the department. She has been working as a midwife with births in hospital, at a birth centre and at home. Ingela is interested in the meaning of childbirth for women's lives. A special focus is women's experiences of giving birth near birth and in a long-term perspective. Further, she is interested in support during childbirth by professionals and non-professionals and the organization of maternity care. Ingela is one of the leaders for a Nordic research network concerning childbirth. She is also representing Sweden (together with Marie Berg) in a COST-network 'Concerns, and consequences: creating a dynamic EU framework for optimal maternity care'. She is involved in projects about homebirth in the Nordic countries, support by professionals and non-professionals, a midwifery model of care in a Nordic context, and doctoral projects in Sweden, Norway and Iceland. Ingela is one of four editors of the Swedish textbook for midwives, *Lärobok för Barnmorskor* and co-editor (with Marie Berg) for *Att stödja och stärka.* Vårdande vid barnafödande (*Support and Strengthen: Caring in Childbearing*).

Holly Powell Kennedy, PhD, CNM, FACNM, FAAN, has been a midwife for 25 years. She is a graduate of the Frontier School of Midwifery & Family Nursing. She obtained her masters degree from the Medical College of Georgia as a family nurse practitioner and her doctoral degree from the University of Rhode Island. She has practised in numerous settings including rural health, community and tertiary hospitals, and in academic practices. She is the Helen Varney Professor of Midwifery at Yale University and President of the American College of Nurse-Midwives. She is on the faculty of King's College London where she was a Fulbright Distinguished Scholar during 2008. Her research includes numerous qualitative studies exploring the work of midwives and its relationship to health outcomes. She has also completed a clinical trial of CenteringPregnancy®, a group model of prenatal care, in two military settings.

Elizabeth (Liz) Smythe, PhD, BA, RM, RGON, is Associate Professor at Auckland University of Technology, New Zealand. She practised as a midwife in the 1980s and then turned to academic interests. She supervises doctoral and masters research from across the health disciplines, but retains a special interest in midwifery. Hermeneutic interpretive phenomenology is her passion. She regularly attends the Institute for Heideggerian Hermeneutical Methodologies founded by Professor Nancy Diekelmann and now led by Associate Professor Pamela Ironside. Alongside her academic career, she is on the International Board of World Vision, concerned with the wellbeing of children from poor backgrounds.

Cheryl Tatano Beck, DNSc, CNM, FAAN, is Board of Trustees Distinguished Professor at the University of Connecticut, School of Nursing. She also has a joint appointment as a Professor in the Department of Obstetrics and Gynecology at the University of Connecticut, School of Medicine. She has received numerous awards, such as the Association of Women's Health, Obstetric, and Neonatal Nursing's Distinguished Professional Service Award, Eastern Nursing Research Society's Distinguished Researcher Award, the Distinguished Alumna Award from Yale University and the Connecticut Nurses' Association's Diamond Jubilee Award for her contribution to nursing research.

Over the past 25 years Cheryl has focused her research efforts on developing a research programme on postpartum mood and anxiety disorders. She has extensively researched these devastating disorders that plague new mothers using both qualitative and quantitative research methods. Based on the findings from her series of qualitative studies, Cheryl has developed the Postpartum Depression Screening Scale (PDSS) which is published by Western Psychological Services.

She is a prolific writer who has published over 125 journal articles on such topics as postpartum depression, postpartum onset of panic disorder, birth trauma, PTSD due to childbirth, phenomenology, grounded theory, meta-analysis, instrument development, meta-synthesis, and narrative analysis. Cheryl is co-author with Dr Denise Polit of the textbook, *Nursing Research: Generating and Assessing Evidence for Nursing Practice.* This text received the 2007 American Journal of Nursing's Book of the Year Award. Cheryl also co-authored with Dr Jeanne Driscoll another book entitled *Postpartum Mood and Anxiety Disorders: A Clinician's Guide* which received the 2006 American Journal of Nursing's Book of the Year Award.

Gill Thomson, PhD, MSc, BSc (Hons), is currently working as a Research Fellow within the Maternal and Infant Nutrition and Nurture Unit (MAINN), School of Health, University of Central Lancashire. Gill has a psychology academic background and has worked within the public, private and voluntary sector. Since completing her Masters in the Psychology of Child Development in 1998, she has been employed on a number of consultation projects, the majority of which involved engaging with vulnerable population groups. Following successful completion of her PhD at the end of 2007 she has been employed by UCLan and has been involved in a number of research/evaluation based projects funded by various Primary Care Trusts to explore biopsychosocial influences and experiences towards maternity services and infant feeding issues. Gill's research interests relate to maternal wellbeing across the peri-natal period, with a particular focus on factors that impact upon the development of attachment relationships. She also has a particular specialism in the interpretive phenomenological based research.

Helena Wigert, PhD, MNSc, RN, is a Senior Lecturer at the Institute of Health and Care Sciences, the Sahlgrenska Academy at University of Gothenburg, Sweden. She is also a clinical Senior Lecturer at Neonatal Intensive Care Unit (NICU), the Queen Silvia Children's Hospital, Sahlgrenska University Hospital, Gothenburg, Sweden. Helena is a paediatric nurse and her research focuses on the caring in NICU for the newborn children and their parents. Her current research projects concern 1) communication between personnel and parents in NICU; and 2) telemedicine with focus communication in neonatal homecare. Helena is also involved in cooperation programme for exchange of students and teachers between Sweden and India. She is author in a Swedish textbook of *Support and Strengthening. Caring in Childbearing;* focusing on family-centred care in NICU.

Foreword

This book is intended for researchers, practitioners, and students to learn about phenomenology as philosophy and method, to see it in action, and consider how to use it in their work. The term 'phenomenon' has many definitions, but there is a common understanding that it is something to be noticed (it is important) and can in some way be known. Our purpose in research is to know things, often with a goal to apply the knowledge. Phenomenology is the study of phenomena – what are those things that should be noticed, and in maternity practice, how can that make a difference in the health of those for whom we care as well as to those who provide the care? It helps us to understand which phenomena are important, and how these phenomena might be very different from our own perceptions. Phenomenology allows us to delve into and listen in on another person's world, and this in turn informs our opinions and learning.

Practitioners struggle with the day-to-day challenge of incorporating scientific evidence into practice. Randomized clinical trials (RCTs) try to limit subjectivity and control context so we can say with more certain assurance that the intervention is the reason for the outcome. Although RCTs have their place, they do not fully reflect the world of the individual experiencing the phenomenon of interest and what is meaningful or relevant to them. Phenomenology is a method that helps us do just that – context is paramount and control loses its power. To understand the levels of complexity of a person's world requires close scrutiny.

This book will help you understand the complexity of phenomenology, including its historical development, philosophical dimensions, and defining characteristics. One of the most important dimensions of phenomenology, regardless of philosopher, is that the world is known and understood contextually and that one person's world can never be fully apprehended by another. As discouraging as that might sound, the authors in this book have artfully portrayed how this actually expands the boundaries of knowing by embracing the contextual and dynamic features of the world in which we live. The first four chapters help you untangle the sometimes confusing terminology and methods of phenomenology which enable you to begin to see how it can be applied to your world. These chapters provide detailed insights into the philosophical underpinnings and methodological applications of descriptive phenomenology (Terese Bondas, Chapter 1), lifeworld phenomenology (Karin Dahlberg, Chapter 2) and interpretive phenomenology (Elizabeth Smythe, Chapter 3). In Chapter 4, Maura Dowling unravels some of the key differences between the various phenomenological approaches, and includes details and references of key phenomenological authors and research in the childbirth and maternity arena. These authors help you to become comfortable with sharing the research process with participants and to realize you do not have to be fully in control and that it all just feels terribly messy at times. That can feel a bit scary, just as it does for the woman who realizes that at some point she needs to surrender to the power of labour. But at the same time it is liberating – in doing so you will get to the knowledge about what is important.

Phenomenology provides a powerful tool to study experiences of health care – each of us is unique and our particular life context influences our needs, responses, and future. The latter chapters help you to see this up close and in action through the articulate voices of study participants as they describe their worlds in which they experienced illness (such as women's lived experiences of pre-eclampsia presented by Joyce Cowan *et al.* in Chapter 6; and a synthesis of phenomenological research into women's experiences of post-partum depression, post-partum onset of panic disorder and post-traumatic stress disorder following childbirth described by Cheryl Tatano Beck in Chapter 11); discrimination (in Chapter 5, Mel Duffy considers the prejudices faced by lesbian women accessing gynaecological services); abandonment (described in the Heideggerian based analysis of women's experiences of a traumatic birth provided by Gill Thomson in Chapter 8); and implications of negative as well as positive care from a parental as well as practitioner-based perspective. In this book the implications and meanings of varying care provision are discussed by Ingela Lundgren in her phenomenological accounts of women's long-term memories of childbirth in Chapter 7 and by Maria Healy, in Chapter 12, who utilized phenomenology to uncover women's experiences of post-natal care in Ireland. In Chapter 9, the research undertaken by Marie Berg and Helena Wigert includes in-depth interviews and observations (with parents and practitioners) to explore parents' experiences of participation in the care of their infant on a neonatal unit. Finally, Lauren Hunter in Chapter 10 offers interpretations of poems written by midwives to explore and illuminate the meanings and experiences of 'being with woman' during childbirth.

Reading phenomenological accounts is not always easy because there is a depth of meaning that can make you squirm when you reflect on your own experiences. Foucault often talked about the 'clinical gaze' that separated the practitioner from the one gazed upon and the power imbalance that follows. Phenomenological writing exposes those gazes and you begin to realize that participant's experiences and perceptions of the intersection of their world with yours may be very different that what you had previously believed. And that is a good thing – because it means that you become more open to their world, cognizant of its reflection of your world, and a better researcher, practitioner, and/or student in the process.

This is a book you will return to again and again as a resource for method and a practical rendering of phenomenology in action. Read it, give it to colleagues to read, and most of all, enjoy it.

Holly Powell Kennedy, October 2010

1 Husserlian phenomenology reflected in caring science childbearing research

Terese Bondas

Introduction

Epistemology is the philosophical branch concerned with the theory of knowledge. Awareness and understanding of the epistemological roots of the method chosen in relation to the topic of interest may enhance the research process, and, ultimately the quality and depth of knowledge that is subsequently developed. The validity of the study may be distorted when the ontological (the conception of reality), and epistemological (nature of knowledge) starting points of the study are not explicated. Likewise, credible evidence for clinical practice suffers if the study is based on incompatible, incorrect or misleading interpretations and secondary or even tertiary references that have been far removed from the primary writings in philosophy, methods or research. A sound philosophical base is important for a discipline, enabling a scientific discussion and critique of the findings. Various methods that have been developed in a phenomenological tradition contribute to basic caring science research and knowledge through accurate and genuine description of phenomena. The overall aim of using a phenomenological perspective is not philosophical in caring science, but the development of knowledge within the disciplinary interest. Giorgi (1985) discusses the difference between a philosophical and a disciplinary knowledge development from the perspective of phenomenology. Thus, phenomenology as a philosophy is here viewed from an epistemological perspective. This provides a foundation for the different phenomenological methods that have been developed in different human science disciplines, and that continue to evolve in these contexts.

The findings from a phenomenological study also direct research in asking new questions, seeing the world through a phenomenological lens and finding phenomena that are relevant and meaningful to caring science. Phenomenology is in tune with caring science as a human science. There is always a perspective in research, otherwise phenomena would not be interesting or meaningful to study within a discipline, as opposed to taking a general once and for all approach across disciplines.

One note of caution: phenomenological methods should not be forced to fit circumstances where they are not appropriate. Unnecessary modifications of methods should not be developed that are inconsistent with phenomenological philosophy (Giorgi 1985). There are many valuable qualitative approaches based on other epistemologies that may be used if modifications are needed. It is not in the interest of science to force one single approach upon every research question.

The imperative of Edmund Husserl, who has been referred to as the father of (modern) phenomenology, is to return to the things themselves (1954/1970). The thing itself is the phenomenon and its structures and essence that are explored in a phenomenological attitude of bracketing previous knowledge, not a natural spontaneous lifeworld attitude. The Husserlian phenomenological foundation is based on constructs such as 'intentionality', 'lifeworld', 'description', and 'epoché'. In this chapter, this foundation is outlined as the epistemological starting point for descriptive phenomenological caring science studies. This is exemplified below by the phenomenological method of Colaizzi (1978) to show one way of developing knowledge of lived experiences in childbearing and care (a pictorial representation of Colaizzi's method is provided in Chapter 11). The phases of deciding on the scope of the study, the aims, the data collection, the phenomenological intuiting and analysing, the reduction or bracketing, and the structure and essence, is described and discussed in relation to the epistemological starting points based on phenomenology. Examples are drawn from a caring science research programme (Bondas-Salonen 1998a,b, Bondas 2000a, Bondas and Eriksson 2001, Bondas 2002, 2005) of women's health and suffering, ante-natal and post-partum care, and the partner's presence during childbearing. Suffering was related to major changes in themselves and their life as a result of illness or violating and inhumane care. A meta-method study of phenomenological method articles and book chapters also emanated from the research programme (Bondas 2000b). The research has continued in the research network BFiN (www.uin.no/bfin) as a programme of qualitative research in evidence-based care, integrating studies and meta-synthesis of childbearing research (cf. Bondas and Hall 2007a,b, Berg *et al.* 2008, Lundgren *et al.* 2009, Wikberg and Bondas 2010).

This chapter uses some of the core ideas of Husserl's phenomenological philosophy and his followers that have developed phenomenological descriptive methods. These ideas serve as a departure to reflect on descriptive phenomenological research and heuristic synthesis in childbearing from a caring science perspective.

The development of Husserlian phemenology and its (mis)use in applied science

Phenomenology as a philosophical movement began with Husserl's extensive writings (Giorgi 1985, Spiegelberg 1975). The history of phenomenology reveals endless variations due to continuous modifications and renewed interpretations, as described by Spiegelberg (1975) in 'The phenomenological movement'. Husserl (1859–1938) developed a philosophy of phenomenology that lends itself to re-interpretation as a strict, rigorous and pure science through description of essential structures of consciousness (Spiegelberg 1975, p. 5). Husserl chose the term 'phenomenology' inspired by his professor of philosophy, Franz Brentano, who emphasized the intentionality of psychic phenomena.

Husserl was worried that human sciences uncritically borrowed its methods from the natural sciences, hence losing connection with people as living human beings (Husserl 1954/1970, p. 17). Husserl's (1954/1970, pp. 3, 17) answer was 'epoché', which means bracketing of the spontaneous attitude to the world, even if the world remains there for us (Husserl 1954/1970, p. 135ff.). Husserl neither denied nor doubted the material, so-called real world. Instead, he argued that all previous knowledge should be bracketed before new knowledge could be brought to the fore:

> Thus I exclude all sciences relating to this natural world no matter how firmly they stand there for me…none is accepted by me; none gives me a foundation…I must not accept such a proposition until after I have put parenthesis around it. That signifies that I may accept such a proposition only in the modified consciousness, the consciousness of judgment-excluding, and therefore not as it is in science, a proposition which claims validity and the validity of which I accept and use.
>
> (Husserl 1954/1970, pp. 61–62)

Husserl was not sure about the creation of knowledge based on the lifeworld; and he described the search for knowledge as 'absolute beginners' (1954/1970, p. 133). Merleau-Ponty (1962) continued this work in relation to the lifeworld and the connection of this concept to that which is experienced by the lived body. Other later phenomenological philosophers, such as Levinás, Ricoeur and Spiegelberg, all added their own nuances to phenomenological philosophy. Subsequent generations of phenomenologists developed methods in pedagogy, psychology and theology through the work of Colaizzi, Giorgi, Moustakas and van Kaam, among others. Duquesne University became the centre for a rich tradition of phenomenological studies. Researchers in human and social sciences, including nursing and caring sciences, could be seen as the fourth generation writing about phenomenological philosophy and applying these phenomenological methods. These researchers had one interest in common: to further a humanistic course of their discipline. Explorations and insights from phenomenology, which began to emerge in the late 1970s and early 1980s in nursing and caring sciences by researchers such as Paterson and Zderad (1976), Oiler (1982), Omery (1983), and Parse (1985), paved the way for experiential issues in childbearing research and phenomenological method applications. The various interpretations of phenomenological philosophy and methods are evident in these early interpreters. However, problems arose because, over time, applied researchers working in this field began to use methods based on mixing primary, secondary and even tertiary references and using other qualitative references that had nothing in common with phenomenology (Bondas 2000b). The critique had been raised already in the 1990s by researchers such as Crotty (1996), Paley (1997), Lawler (1998), and Porter (1998), among others. The recent development of meta-method in meta-synthesis (Paterson *et al.* 2001, Bondas and Hall 2007a,b) also confirms a mixed language use and methodological praxis in phenomenological studies. Phenomenological research has also been mixed with the methodological language and practice of grounded theory, ethnography and other qualitative descriptive studies. In some of the studies, the researcher's theoretical, clinical and/or his or her own lifeworld perspectives seem to dominate. The researcher has not accomplished the phenomenological task: deciding the phenomenon of interest for the study and uncovering the lived experience of the participating persons. In other studies, the research does not go beyond a thematic analysis; the essence of the phenomenon is not illuminated, or the challenge might not even have been recognized (cf. Bondas 2000b, Paterson *et al.* 2001, Bondas and Hall 2007a,b, Sandelowski and Barroso 2007).

In nursing and caring science literature, there are even different views of phenomenology as: a philosophy, a variety of philosophies, science, theory, method(s), modified methods and combined with an ontological position as lifeworld-led care and an attitude to life and care (Bondas 2000a,b). Phenomenology may be seen as an umbrella concept, and thus, the specific basis that is being used in any particular circumstance always needs to be explicated when this approach is used in writings and research.

What a phenomenological Husserlian epistemology can offer caring science childbearing research

The Husserlian foundation includes phenomenological constructs such as 'phenomenon' and 'intentionality', 'lifeworld' 'bracketing', 'description' and 'structure' and 'essence', among others. These will be outlined in relation to the caring science research programme of Bondas that employed Colaizzi's descriptive phenomenological method, based on Husserl's philosophy.

Phenomenon and intentionality

Husserl used the word phenomenon to denominate that which emerges in consciousness when we think, experience or imagine whether it exists in reality. In a study, this intuitive knowledge is data ('inside-knowledge') which appears in an immediate situation when collecting the data with the participant in the study. In Mohanty's (1987) words it is not a question of photographical resemblance: the phenomenon as revealed by the speaker is not necessarily the same as that seen by the observer. Understanding of the phenomena appears as it is given in the realm of the person's lifeworld which exists before interpretations or explanations. The intentionality of human consciousness is the primary phenomenological lens through which we view our lifeworld:

> Consciousness is considered to be the principal realm since anything whatsoever that we can know or speak about must come through consciousness.
>
> (Giorgi 1983, p. 134)

Intentional consciousness means that intentional objects do not necessarily exist, but when a person describes what s/he remembers, s/he refers to something that evokes an intentional phenomenological structure (Giorgi 1983). The meaning of time from a phenomenological perspective is the lived time in the person's unique lifeworld. The tempus of existence, that what once was, is and will be, is not differentiated but clustered together. A person may simultaneously think about what happened in an existing moment while also anticipating what will happen. The past exists in memories and the future through expectations. Both exist through intentionality in the existing moment.

Finding a phenomenon may be the most difficult endeavour for the novice as well as the seasoned researcher when the gaze easily remains narrowed by the researcher's lifeworld. These pre-conceptions include theoretical knowledge as well as personal and/or clinical knowledge. The interest of phenomenology in all its variations lies in the knowledge of phenomena based on lived experiences, which in turn may have an impact on understanding and development of care from a caring science perspective. Childbearing includes human experiences in all its variety, and deeply touches matters of life and death, health and suffering. The caring science interests are in line with the ideas of Husserl, who expressed his worry over the state of the natural sciences:

> fact-minded sciences make merely fact-minded people
>
> (Husserl 1954/1970, p. 6)

Research based on the natural sciences has created disciplines that exclude all value positions, all questions of reason or unreason of their human subject matter and its cultural configurations. Husserl wondered if the world and human existence could have any meaning for life if the sciences only recognize truth as being objectively established. He thus offered phenomenology as a cure for what he saw as the 'crisis' of science, which had lost its meaning for life (1954/1970, p. 5).

Finding phenomena for a childbirth research programme in caring science

The core interests of caring science are closely related to caring and values, and the discipline of phenomenology suits caring science research well. It offers a human science discipline with its task to create knowledge of caring that has the potential to alleviate human suffering and promote health

(Eriksson 2006). The worldview in this chapter sees caring science as an open and autonomous human science discipline that has its own ontological and theoretical core, and which creates knowledge based on its own basic motives. It takes an ethical attitude which values the primacy of human dignity, in which practitioners take responsibility for their life and for that of others and which includes their will to minister and to be there for one another (Eriksson 2006). Human beings reflect on their health in existential boundary situations, such as giving birth to a baby (Bondas 2000a, 2005). In maternal care research phenomena of existential suffering or health are limited (insights into women's experiences of traumatic/difficult births and post-partum mood and anxiety disorders are presented in Chapters 7, 8 and 11). Instead, the research has focused on motherhood, maternal role and identity, crisis and stress, and symptoms. It is important to understand phenomena in childbearing to promote the woman's and the whole family's health and alleviate suffering. It is also important to understand that new motherhood requires the woman to care for the new baby as well as herself when she is recovering from a difficult delivery or operative procedures.

An approach that is based on ideas from Husserlian phenomenology offers a lived perspective to guide the search for phenomena. It may start with the interplay between existing knowledge, one's own research interests and one's own and others' experiences as illuminated in storytelling, media and art picturing childbirth. (Refer to Beck (Chapter 11) for a further example of research utilising a Husserlian approach). Husserlian-based phenomenology develops knowledge of phenomena, and not any experience *per se*. Finding the phenomena is therefore important and a prerequisite for research in this tradition. The phenomena that were chosen in my childbirth research programme (Bondas 2000a, 2005) were not to be found in the scientific literature and had been overlooked in the health care information to childbearing families. The phenomenological research process starts in silence and peace to be able to concentrate on the phenomenon. Preparations emerge in the mood of openness to the phenomenon that has been decided on, whilst also making concrete decisions on the design and implementation of the study. Phenomena in my research programme (Bondas 2000a, 2005) emerged from personal experiences based on my own childbirth experiences as mother and professional, art and movies, clinical experiences, talking to female as well as male acquaintances, and a comprehensive knowledge of the research area and theories in this particular field. Selecting the familiar is natural; however, it is easier to be open minded and curious in relation to unfamiliar phenomena. After my first study was completed I found that each subsequent study brought new phenomena to inform and understand the lived experiences of childbearing women.

The primary aim of my resulting caring science phenomenological research programme was to describe women's lived experiences of pregnancy, antenatal and post-partum care, and the presence of the partner at the birth of the baby. The second aim was to integrate all the phenomenological studies

I undertook into a heuristic synthesis. This synthesis represents a creative leap from the phenomenological findings of the studies in the research programme combined with previous research and the caring science perspective inspired by Moustakas (1990, 1994) and Morse (1997). The rationale was to provide qualitative evidence-based knowledge for care from the pregnant women's and the new mothers' lifeworld as well as contributions to caring science disciplinary knowledge. I also wished to heighten societal consciousness and increase reflections in parents-to-be and new parents, friends and extended families about women's experiences in childbearing. The five research questions that underpinned the programme were: 1) What are women's lived experiences of pregnancy? (Bondas and Eriksson 2001); 2) What are women's lived experiences of antenatal care? (Bondas 2002); 3) What are women's lived experiences of post-partum care? (Bondas-Salonen 1998b); 4) What are women's lived experiences of the partner's presence at the birth of their baby? (Bondas-Salonen 1998a); and 5) What is the heuristic synthesis of the four phenomenological studies in relation to caring science and previous research? (Bondas 2000a, 2005).

Lifeworld knowledge

Husserl (1954/1970) was first to outline the construct 'lifeworld' (German construct 'lebenswelt'). The lifeworld is the foundation of knowledge, and Husserl described the lifeworld as a nourishing soil and support, rather than a logical ground (1954/1970, pp. 18, 131). Lifeworld is always there before science (p. 33); a 'prescientific lifeworld' (p. 43) and forms the fundamental basis for meaning in the scientific endeavour, even for the natural sciences (p. 48). The empirically intuited surrounding world has, of necessity, an empirical style according to Husserl (1954/1970, p. 31). He discussed our ability to make fantasies of the world as it could be but only in relation to the style that we know. The only real world is the one that is actually given through perception, and which is ever experienced; this is our everyday lifeworld (Husserl 1954/1970, p. 49). 'While present time is given us directly, past and future times appear to us only indirectly by way of our present representations of ourselves as experiencing the past or as experiencing the future object' (Husserl 1954/1970, p. 40). The contrast between the subjectivity of the lifeworld and the objective, 'the true' world lies in the fact that the latter is a theoretical-logical construction. The lifeworld is distinguished in all respects precisely by it being experiencable. The lifeworld is a realm of original self-evidence 'the thing itself' in immediate presence, in memory, in intuition (Husserl 1954/1970, p. 128). (Also refer to Chapter 2 for detailed insights into lifeworld phenomenology.)

Expressing the lifeworld in the childbirth research programme

Only those who have experienced the phenomena of interest, and are willing to describe their experiences should be invited to participate in a phenomenological study (Colaizzi 1978, Giorgi 1975, 1985, Hycner 1985, Moustakas 1994). According to Colaizzi (1978) it is not possible to give recommendations about how many persons should participate in a study. It is a decision that is made separately in every study when no new insights or new themes emerge from the findings. The background data will highlight the differences in the actual research programme, for example age and parity between the participants. However this data is not used for comparison in a phenomenological study. Writing a research diary is of uttermost importance in a phenomenological study, to include reflections on previous writings and thoughts. There are specific recommendations for data collection connected to the different phenomenological methods. The data as collected from the participants is only one aspect of the lifeworld. Data collection is a dialectical exchange between the researcher and the participant in a particular lifeworld situation. There is no manipulation or use of data that has been collected for other purposes (Giorgi 1975). The phenomenological interview starts preferably with an open question: 'What was your experience...?' The interview situation is flexible and the researcher decides when to ask clarifying questions. The interview ends when the participant has nothing more to tell, normally signalled by a period of silence. After this time one last question is posed: 'is there anything that you would like to add?' New data may be collected by looking back or by looking forward, describing hopes, dreams and wishes.

In the research programme undertaken by Bondas, nine women were originally recruited, who were followed from pregnancy to two-and-a-half years after delivery. In addition, non-participant observations of care situations and dialogical interviews were undertaken during three months (31 women). A schedule for sensitizing dialogical interviews based on prior observations of relevant maternity care situations was developed to collect data (Bondas 2000a; Bondas 2005); an approach endorsed by Colaizzi (1978).

Bracketing

Husserl (1954/1970) provides the primary phenomenological answer, an imperative to go back to the things themselves:

> We parenthesize everything which that positing encompasses with respect to being: thus the whole natural world which is continually 'there for us', 'on hand', and which will always remain there according to consciousness as an 'actuality' even if we choose to parenthesize it.
> (Husserl 1954/1970, pp. 61–62)

Husserl refers to this as the 'epoché'; a withholding of natural naive validities – in respect to all objective sciences in regard to all objective theoretical interest' (Husserl 1954/1970, p. 133).

He further states:

Thus I exclude all sciences relating to this natural world no matter how firmly they stand there for me…none is accepted by me; none gives me a foundation…I must not accept such a proposition until after I have put parenthesis around it…'

(Husserl 1954/1970, pp. 61–62)

Spiegelberg (1975) differentiates between those who accepted Husserl's transcendental phenomenology based on the idea of an absolutely pure consciousness and those who did not. The critics point out that Husserl not only strived for eidetic reduction (i.e. bracketing the intentionality), but that consciousness itself should pass a transcendental reduction, becoming essences of structures without the need for human existence (Bengtsson 1988). Husserl's transcendental approach has been criticized as ultra-positivism, a universal phenomenology of essences that lacks connection to human beings. Yet, the phenomena are the focus in the phenomenology of Husserl; how phenomena appear for a person in his or her lifeworld. Merleau-Ponty (1962, p. xv) stresses the point that the critique towards Husserl is erroneous, and that Husserl did not separate essence and existence but instead the essence in a Husserlian sense is to: 'bring back all the living relationships of experience, as the fisherman's net'. Bracketing is further explicated: 'it slackens the intentional threads which attach us to the world and thus brings them to our notice' (Merleau-Ponty 1962, p. xiii). 'Absolutism is fooling oneself and is not possible' (Spiegelberg 1975, p. xxiv).

Bracketing in the research programme

Bracketing in the research programme was a critical, careful exploration that required probing of phenomena by using questioning doubt, enough data, free variation, and an epistemological humbleness. It is a dynamic awareness more than an extinction of the previous knowledge and the lifeworld of the researcher. Personal and professional experiences combined with the scientific knowledge facilitate, but can also impede the phenomenological research process through partial prejudiced perspectives. One example was my own positive view of the body in pregnancy that had to be modified in the encounters of women's descriptions of their experiences. I met participating pregnant women that described how they hated their pregnant body and how their weight gain and their enlarging belly disgusted them. They used metaphors such as 'elephants' or 'toads' (Bondas 2000a; Bondas and Eriksson 2001). I had to be open for the phenomenon, and reflect on my pre-knowledge, attitude and questions in the interviews and analysis. Bracketing may be handled by reading, writing and intuiting during the whole process. Reflecting and writing a research diary has been helpful in my research programme as it is not possible to complete bracketing as a task in the beginning of the study. The striving was to explore phenomena as they appeared in the consciousness of the participating women: to reach the phenomena through the experiences that were described in the interviews and situations of care. Time was set aside for data collection and continuous phenomenological intuiting, analysing and writing. Time was needed for reading and doing phenomenology. Bracketing was an ongoing, conscious process in order to maintain the focus on the phenomena in the complex world of childbearing and my everyday life. The question was never about what actually had taken place or not. The focus was the lived experiences of the participating women.

Phenomenological description

The phenomenological method of Colaizzi as applied within my research programme (Bondas 2000a, 2005) was based on the Husserlian description: 'I seek not to instruct but to lead, to point out and describe what I see' (1954/1970, p. 18). Phenomena were to be described as they were experienced from women's consciousness. Husserl posits that each of us has our own perspective, and each of these perspectives count. Expressions made by people about a phenomenon are not in themselves literal descriptions of that phenomenon, but may be used as a kind of proxy description as they refer to phenomena from an inside perspective (Husserl 1954/1970, p. 28). Mohanty (1987, p. 43), an American phenomenological philosopher, explicates the research work of description: 'It follows that the task of describing does not necessarily exclude the exercise of thought, the practice of analysis, the activity of reflection.' Phenomenology is description, not construction or creation (Merleau-Ponty 1962, p. x). Husserlian-based phenomenological research may metaphorically be seen as a strained intuitive watching and waiting, during which description is carried out in an archaeological attitude that combines humility of the observer, and awareness of the complexity of phenomena (Spiegelberg 1975). Phenomenological description is not a deductive system, not a hypothetical confirming or non-confirming system. It is not an approach that constructs interpretative frames of reference or theoretical models, it is not reconstructive, and it is not an analysis which would seek conditions or an explanation system (Giorgi 1989). The position of the data is always primary, and data are never collected to provide evidence for existing theoretical constructions (Giorgi 1992).

Colaizzi (1978) argues that recorded verbal data should be transcribed, and that it is important to listen to the tapes, to try to understand their content as a whole, and to become familiar with the data. Expressions are noted, and reflected upon, and the meanings are formulated. Then a naming takes place. This is a thematization of the meaning units. It is not based on counting or tallying the occurrence of meaning units in the data. Moustakas (1994, p. 180) uses the term 'horizonalization' for the Husserlian equal value to illuminate the focus on description of the phenomenon of the study. Themes are grouped with other themes that share meaning content, and this process is then used to create clusters. These clusters are then validated in relation to the original expressions and meaning units. An exhaustive description that reflects the variation in the text is created, and an essential structure is formulated. The process whereby an understanding of the phenomenology and the research area is achieved, while bracketing presuppositions in a research diary written throughout the research process, is outlined in Figure 1.1.

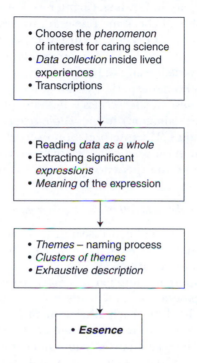

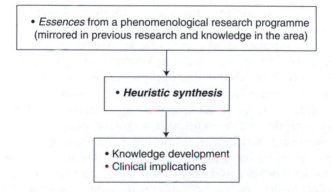

Figure 1.1 Phenomenological descriptive study: from essence to essences in heuristic synthesis of a phenomenological research programme

Colaizzi recommends that participants should be perceived as 'co-research-ers' and that validation should be undertaken with the participants in the study. Beck *et al.* (1994) compared differences in validity between the phe-nomenological methods of Colaizzi, Giorgi and van Kaam, and stated that the differences are technical. However, they are all developed in the descriptive Duquesne tradition (refer to Dowling, Chapter 4). Van Kaam (1959) recom-mends that experts should check the research process. Giorgi (1975, 1983, 1985, 1989) notes that if all experts are in favour, everyone may be wrong and then the judgement used becomes empirical and not phenomenologi-cal. Free imaginative variation and reduction always includes the perspective of the other person who has experienced the phenomenon in question. In this way of seeing, the use of a few critics is not enough: the work should be exposed (through dissemination) to the whole scientific community to be the judge of the findings. The interpretation exceeds the views of the par-ticipants and the theoretical perspective is not an every-day perspective. The participants know their own experience but not the experience of others.

Description as applied to the childbirth research programme

The phenomena in my childbirth research programme were studied as they presented themselves as lived experiences in the consciousness of the participants. I did not deny other ontological views of the world but my phenomenological approach implied a preference to study childbearing women's lifeworld experiences and to describe them. The lived experi-ences are described by the participating women from the perspective of their unique lifeworld, and these descriptions are the data for the phenom-enological analysis. The data analysis required a continuous bracketing of pre-knowledge. The essential structure and variations based in the exhaus-tive descriptions was intended to capture the phenomena of pregnancy, antenatal care, partner's presence at the birth of the baby, and post-partum care from the perspective of women, who have lived through these experi-ences. The findings may be directly transferred to evidence-based care as a departure for innovations in caring and for parents-to-be to mirror their own experiences. In my childbearing research project (Bondas 2000a), the participants were offered the opportunity to read their transcribed interviews. The longitudinal nature of the interviews also enabled clarifica-tion. Two of the participants took up the opportunity to read the findings, which they agreed to be resonant with their own experiences. These par-ticipants were surprised by and grateful for the findings. They reported that it was a relief to recognize that they were not alone in their experi-ences. Nurses, midwives and doctors in the participating units evaluated the findings. There were defensive comments regarding the women's negative and condemning experiences of care-givers. They doubted not only the participating women's experiences, they also doubted phenomenological research. However, I have subsequently met midwives and other care-givers, who have remodelled their care based on insights from the findings of my research programme.

Knowledge: structure and essences

Knowledge is acquired through detailed analysis and careful description under-taken in a phenomenological attitude of bracketing previous knowledge and intuition expressed in structures and essence (Giorgi 1975, Spiegelberg 1975, 1982). Husserl (1948/1973, p. 341) argues for the importance of essences:

> It then becomes evident that a unity runs through this multiplicity of successive figures, that in such free variations of an original image, e.g. of a thing, an invariant is necessarily retained as the necessary general form without which an object such as this thing, as an example of this kind, would not be thinkable at all (if this inner core changes, then it is another object).
>
> (Husserl 1948/1973, p. 341)

Essence is the basic characteristic or distinctive feature of phenomena reached through imagining and variation of an experience. Essences are never exhaustive and access to consciousness is always inadequate (Moustakas 1994). The difference between a phenomenological philosophical univer-sal essence and a disciplinary essence is the cultural and social limitation belonging to human sciences that create their own perspectives (Giorgi 1985, 1989). The perspective includes that which is interesting and relevant for the actual discipline. Obtaining essential insights requires that we decide what the necessary characteristics are and that which is an accidental occurrence. The phenomenology of appearances is watching and listening to modes of appearance of the phenomenon; not just what is expressed, but how it is expressed. It is seeing the same phenomenon in different ways that unveils something fundamental. Spiegelberg (1975) exemplifies this through the example of how art may look different in different light conditions.

Knowledge in the childbirth research programme

An example of an essential structure found in my research programme was 'postpartum care as rest and learning in communion' (Bondas-Salonen 1998b, Bondas 2000a). The transitional process from being an expectant mother to being a new mother occurs slowly but intensely with unique expressions during the first days after the baby is born. The child's wellbeing becomes her first concern and she wants to share her new life situation with her family against the background of her past and present, and the family's shared future. Caring during post-partum is experienced as confirmatory moments of communion which she recognizes all the more starkly in the light of her experiences of absence of caring. The new mother experiences caring in sharing her new life situation with the midwife; learning directly through the midwife's teaching and indirectly when the midwife is at hand but enables the woman to be in peace and quiet with the baby and the family that she defines. Other new mothers care for the woman reciprocally, through sharing the same situation, helping each other and learning to care for the baby, themselves, and their family.

Heuristic synthesis

Phenomenological studies may be integrated through the application of heuristic synthesis. Heuristic synthesis was developed in the research programme (Bondas 2000a, 2005) as a methodological device to combine the findings of several Husserlian-based phenomenological studies. The interest is to create an essence of several essences of interconnected phenomena. Webster (1989, p. 667) defines heuristics as: 'serving to indicate or point out, stimulating interest as a means of furthering investigation'. The roots are in the Greek word 'heuriskein', which means to find out or discover. Webster (1989, p. 1443) defines 'synthesis' as 'the combining of the constituent elements or separate material or abstract entities into a single or unified entity', and 'a complex whole formed by combining'. It is the opposite of analysis, dividing into parts. Heuristic synthesis is thus discovery through combining of constituting elements, which are the findings of different studies in the research programme of phenomenological studies. (Further examples of synthesized phenomenological findings are presented in Chapters 7, 9 and 11.)

Synthesis in the research programme

As noted above, in the research programme, a heuristic synthesis based on four different phenomenological studies of childbearing and care was developed (Bondas 2005). The essence of the essences of the findings in different studies was first intuited and analysed, and then compared to previous research and theories. The synthesis may metaphorically be viewed as a thick rope made of different colours and fabrics. The different parts of the material create the rope; at the same time the individual threads may be seen and can be drawn apart. The phenomenological essence and structure plays the leading role and the merger with theory is not a question of adaptation or forcing. The synthesis in the case of this programme was an extension of the descriptive method of Colaizzi (1978).

The heuristic synthesis in the research programme united the time period of childbearing through the tapestry of health, suffering and communion in the metaphor 'being *with* child' (Bondas 2000a, 2005). Starting from the day the woman begins to plan and wish for a baby that imaginary child becomes part of her lifeworld. The child will always be a part of her, sometimes close, sometimes far away because of the circumstances and experiences in her life. When the woman, even in her imagination, loses the child she becomes separated from dreams, expectations and plans in lost possibilities and lost joy. It is not any child but her and her partner's perfect baby in their family. The changes in existence; bodily changes, variations in mood, ill health that is considered part of pregnancy and worries, health promotion, health consciousness and healthy behaviour continue in the pains and worries of the birth. The transformation into joy or deeper worry continues in the paradoxical post-partum existence of uncertainty and loneliness, although there is joy when everything has turned out right. Women share the life and health changes in being *with* child in family communion, communion with others in childbearing, sisterly communion and caring communion with the midwife and other professional carers (Bondas 2000a, 2005). The questions she asks, and her constant need to tell her childbirth story may be seen as purging when there is an experience of communion for the woman. The woman may feel how listening takes away, 'rinses' and alleviates her suffering, which may be hidden in language, humour and self-ironic comments to maintain her dignity if the other person, especially in professional care, does not recognize her suffering, or avoids or overlooks it. The motive and starting point for care are in the lifeworlds of the woman, the father to be and her family in childbearing. Implications for development of professional care emerge from the evidence of the phenomenological research programme (Bondas 2000a, 2005). Figure 1.1 on page 11 depicted the research process in a descriptive phenomenological study to a heuristic synthesis in a phenomenological research programme.

Final reflections

It can be argued that the current focus in science in the health services has moved from finding out what is really going on ('doing the right thing') to a focus on the correct methods of doing research, without necessarily being concerned about whether what is being found is useful and/or meaningful ('doing things right'). There is no simple formula in science and the discussion is on-going. Phenomenological methods offer a systematic, rigorous and critical means to study human experiences from a caring science perspective in childbearing research. However, the development of these methods has been slow. This is a concern, as there are complex dynamic phenomena in childbearing from a lifeworld perspective that are not captured by the methods developed in other disciplines that take a 'normal science' perspective. Another challenge for the phenomenological researcher is to find the phenomena that matter to the participants, when the caring science researcher carries a perspective from her/his clinical practice and previous theory laden conceptualizations. The source of phenomenological knowledge is the experiencing person and an epistemology of their specific lifeworld. Recognizing this means that phenomenological designs may open up new perspectives and develop childbirth care based on the lived experiences of the woman, her partner and their family members.

In conclusion, the following are the basic assumptions of phenomenological research from a caring science perspective:

* Phenomenological research is based on phenomenological epistemology and employs methodological rules that may vary across different phenomenological approaches.
* Phenomenological research requires study of and insights into the ideas of phenomenological philosophy.
* Phenomenological research requires a reflective, systematic, and thoughtful application of the chosen phenomenological method.
* Rich knowledge from a lifeworld perspective can be attained through Husserlian-based phenomenological descriptive methods.
* Phenomenology may as an epistemology and methodology contribute to caring science research and knowledge through genuine description of phenomena.
* A heuristic synthesis of phenomenological studies may be developed through a creative leap integrating different studies from a caring science perspective using the heuristic phenomenological method.

Conclusion

Phenomenological Husserlian research in childbearing may illuminate women's and other family members' lifeworld, including their expectations, fears and wishes for childbirth, the baby and care. It has the potential to develop new caring science knowledge that has direct evidence for clinical caring practice. Phenomenological research has the potential to challenge previous knowledge and practice in antenatal, birth and post-partum care. Heuristic synthesis from a phenomenological perspective is a meta-method endeavour. It has been developed to create an essence of essences that connect several phenomenological studies into one phenomenological research programme, just as expectations of childbirth, pregnancy, birth and post-partum create an interconnected experiential period: 'to be *with* child' (Bondas 2000a, 2005).

References

Beck C.T., Keddy B.A. and Cohen M.Z. (1994) Reliability and validity issues in phenomenological research. *Western Journal of Nursing Research* 16, 3, 254–267.

Bengtsson J. (1988) *Sammanflätningar. Fenomenologi från Husserl till Merleau-Ponty.* (in Swedish) *Phenomenology. From Husserl to Merleau Ponty.* Daidalos, Göteborg.

Berg M., Bondas T., Hall E., Lundgren I., Olafsdottir O., Støre Brinchmann B. and Vehviläinen-Julkunen K. (2008) Evidence based care and childbearing – A critical approach. *International Journal of Qualitative Studies on Health and Wellbeing* 3, 239–247.

Bondas T. (2000a) *Att vara med barn: en vårdvetenskaplig studie av kvinnors upplevelser under perinatal tid.* (in Swedish) *To be with child: a caring science study of women's perinatal experiences.* Doctoral diss. (Summary in English). Åbo Akademi University: Åbo.

Bondas T. (2000b) Hur presenteras fenomenologiska närmelsesätt i vårdvetenskaplig metodlitteratur? (in Swedish) How are phenomenological approaches described in caring science method literature? In *Proceedings VI. Kansallinen hoitotieteellinen konferenssi 29–30.9.2000, Hoitotieteellisen tutkimuksen ydinkysymyksiä terveyden edistämisessä perusterveydenhuollossa ja erikoissairaanhoidossa.* Kuopio University Reports E: Social Sciences 19, Kuopio, Finland, 44–50.

Bondas T. (2002) Finnish women's experiences of antenatal care. *Midwifery* 18, 61–71.

Bondas T. (2005) To be with child: a heuristic synthesis in maternal care. In *Trends in Midwifery Research* (Balin, R. ed.), 119–136, Nova Science: New York.

Bondas T. and Eriksson K. (2001) Women's lived experiences of pregnancy – a tapestry of health and suffering. *Qualitative Health Research* 11, 824–840.

Bondas T. and Hall E. (2007a) Challenges in the approaches to metasynthesis research. *Qualitative Health Research* 17, 113–121.

Bondas T. and Hall E. (2007b) A decade of metasynthesis research: A meta-method study. *International Journal of Qualitative Studies on Health and Wellbeing* 2 (2), 101–113.

Bondas-Salonen T. (1998a) How women experience the presence of their partners at the birth of their baby. *Qualitative Health Research* 8, 784–800.

Bondas-Salonen T. (1998b) New mothers' experiences of postpartum care – a phenomenological follow-up study. *Journal of Clinical Nursing* 7, 165–174.

Colaizzi P.F. (1978) Psychological research as the phenomenologist views it. In *Existential–Phenomenological Alternatives for Psychology.* (In Valle R.S. and King M. eds), Oxford University Press: New York.

Crotty M. (1996) *Phenomenology and Nursing Research.* Churchill Livingstone: Melbourne.

Eriksson K. (2006) *The Suffering Human Being.* Nordic Studies Press: Chicago.

Giorgi A. (1975) An application of the phenomenological method in psychology. In *Duquesne Studies in Phenomenological Psychology, Vol 2* (Giorgi A., Fisher C.T. and Murray, E.L. eds), 82–103, Duquesne University Press: Pittsburgh.

Giorgi A. (1983) Concerning the possibility of phenomenological psychological research. *Journal of Phenomenological Psychology* 14, 2, 129–169.

Giorgi A. (ed.) (1985) *Phenomenology and Psychological Research.* Duquesne University Press: Pittsburgh.

Giorgi A. (1989) One type of analysis of descriptive data: Procedures involved in following a scientific phenomenological method. *Methods* 1, 3, 39–61.

Giorgi A. (1992) Description versus interpretation: Competing alternative strategies for qualitative research, *Journal of Phenomenological Psychology* 23, 2, 119–135.

Husserl E. (1954/1970) *The Crisis of European Sciences and transcendental phenomenology.* Northwestern University Press: Evanston.

Husserl E. (1948/1973) *Experience and judgement.* Northwestern University Press: Evanston.

Hycner R.H. (1985) Some guidelines for the phenomenological analysis of interview data. *Human Studies* 8, 279–303.

Lawler J. (1998) Phenomenologies as research methodologies for nursing: From philosophy to researching practice. *Nursing Inquiry* 5, 104–111.

Lundgren I., Karlsdottir S.I. and Bondas T. (2009) Long-time memories and experiences of childbirth in a Nordic context – a secondary analysis. *International Journal of Qualitative Studies on Health and Wellbeing* 4, 115–128.

Merleau-Ponty M. (1962) *Phenomenology of perception.* Routledge & Kegan Paul: London.
Mohanty J.N. (1987) Philosophical description and descriptive philosophy. In *Phenomenology: Descriptive or Hermeneutic.* The first Annual Symposium of the Simon Silverman Phenomenology Centre. Duquesne University Press: Pittsburgh.
Morse J.M. (1997) Considering theory derived from qualitative research. In *Completing a qualitative project: Details and dialogue.* (Morse J.M. ed.), 163–189. Sage: Thousand Oaks.
Moustakas C. (1990) *Heuristic Research: Design, Methodology, and Applications.* Sage: Newbury Park.
Moustakas C. (1994) *Phenomenological Research Methods.* Sage: Thousand Oaks.
Oiler C. (1982) The phenomenological approach in nursing research. *Nursing Research* 31, 3, 178–181.
Omery A. (1983) Phenomenology: a method for nursing. *Advances in Nursing Science* 1, 49–63.
Paley J. (1997) Husserl, phenomenology and nursing. *Journal of Advanced Nursing* 26, 187–193.
Parse R.R. (1985) The phenomenological method. In *Nursing Research: Qualitative methods* (Parse R.R., Coyne A.B. and Smith M.J. eds), 15–26. Prentice Hall: Bowie.
Paterson J. and Zderad L. (1976) *Humanistic Nursing.* Wiley: New York.
Paterson B., Thorne S.E., Canam C. and Jillings C. (2001) *Meta-study of Qualitative Health Research: A Practical Guide to Meta-analysis and Meta-synthesis.* Sage: Thousand Oaks.
Porter E.J. (1998) On 'being inspired' by Husserl's phenomenology: reflections on Omery's exposition of methods in nursing. *Advances in Nursing Science* 21, 1, 16–28.
Sandelowski M. and Barroso J. (2007) *Handbook for Synthesizing Qualitative Research.* Springer: New York.
Spiegelberg H. (1975) *Doing Phenomenology: Essays on and in Phenomenology.* Martinus Nijhoff: The Hague.
van Kaam A. (1959) Phenomenal analysis: Exemplified by a study of the experience of really feeling understood. *Journal of Individual Psychology* 15, 66–72.
Webster (1989) *Encyclopedic Unabridged Dictionary of the English Language.* Gramercy, New York.
Wikberg A. and Bondas T. (2010) A patient perspective in research on intercultural caring in maternity care: A meta-ethnography. *International Journal of Qualitative Studies on Health and Wellbeing* 5, 1–15.

Further reading

Giorgi A. (1970) *Psychology as a Human Science: A Phenomenologically-based Approach.* Harper and Row: New York.
Giorgi A. (1971) Phenomenology and experimental psychology. In *Duquesne Studies in phenomenological psychology, Vol 1* (Giorgi A., Fischer W.F. and von Eckartsberg R. eds), 6–16, Duquesne University Press: Pittsburgh.
Husserl E. (1913/1982) *Ideas Pertaining to a Pure Phenomenology and to a Phenomenological Philosophy – First Book: General Introduction to a Pure Phenomenology. Collected Works: Volume 2.* Nijhoff: The Hague.
Spiegelberg H. (1982) *The Phenomenological Movement: A Historical Introduction.* (3rd rev. ed.), Martinus Nijhoff: The Hague.

2 Lifeworld phenomenology for caring and health care research

Karin Dahlberg

Introduction

After one decade of the new millennium, we see new and successful treatments of diseases that previously were incurable. We also see that people in Western society die older now than before, and we see that mothers and babies in our countries survive childbearing and birth to a greater extent than ever. While many of these improvements are due to medical innovations and care, there are also negative consequences. Human conditions, which previously were not understood as diseases, are now described as pathological phenomena, are categorized, given diagnoses and are medically treated. Medicine's approach to childbearing, birthing and motherhood is such an example.

This situation could be acceptable if other problematic aspects of modern medicine were not evident. Medicine, as a branch of modern science, adopted a mechanistic world view early on that describes the human being as a machine, certainly complex, but still a thing among other things that can be thoroughly understood piece by piece. Mathematics became the solution to all scientific questions. Only the biomedical aspects of a person that could be measured and quantified were considered scientific enough and consequently all immeasurable aspects, such those that belong to one's mind, thoughts, feelings, wishes, intentions and other existential phenomena, were left outside of the scientific domain. The consequent dualistic approach to health care led to the prevalent view that mind and body should be studied, understood and treated separately.

By obeying the rules of modern science it can be argued that we have become blind and remote to what life is, what humans are and what the meaning of life and existence is.

> Few things in the human world are as natural and obvious as birth and death. Nevertheless, these aspects of life have become artificial and foreign, and health care generally has come to treat them, like much in contemporary medicine, as merely technical processes.
>
> (Dahlberg *et al.* 1999, p. 215)

This quotation belongs to a critical commentary on a study of routine amniotomy as a component of active management of labour. In modern health care, childbearing and birthing have become medical events that usually take place in a technical context associated with diseases and pharmacological treatment (hospital) (see also Thomson, Chapter 8).

I do not want to throw out the baby with the bath water. I believe that there are many good and important aspects of medicine that are of crucial import for the understanding of childbearing and birthing, and which support the health of mothers, fathers and babies. I want health care to save this knowledge, but I want to throw out the dirty water of too much technologization, categorization and medicalization, which has developed beyond any reasonable limits, and, instead, pour in the fresh water of an approach to health care science and research that is based in lifeworld phenomenology.

The aim of this chapter is to outline some essential features of lifeworld phenomenology and relate them to a) the care that is the context of childbearing and birthing, and b) the scientific enquiry of childbearing and birthing. I build on my experiences from phenomenologically based research, which has both empirical and philosophical strands.[1]

Lifeworld phenomenology

The philosophical idea of the lifeworld was introduced by Husserl (1970/1936) whose intent was for lifeworld theory to become the new basis for all scientific understanding of humans. In particular, the lifeworld theory is essential to phenomenology, which begins within the lifeworld as our lived, but often disregarded, existence in the world.

The lifeworld theory was further explicated by Merleau-Ponty, who expresses the idea of lifeworld as our 'being to the world'. His poetic description of the notion of lifeworld is often cited:

> To return to the things themselves is to return to that world which precedes knowledge, of which knowledge always *speaks*, and in relation to which every scientific schematization is an abstract and derivative sign language, as is geography in relation to the countryside in which we have learnt beforehand what a forest, a prairie or a river is.
>
> (Merleau-Ponty 1995/1945, p. ix)

A phenomenological message is that we live in and through the lifeworld, and that we actually can never escape this complex, meaning filled and lived reality that is there for us whatever we do, whether that is caring or researching. The lifeworld is pre-scientific, pre-theoretical and pre-reflective, which means that we cannot judge about anything in our world other than in relation to our experience of it, always in the midst of the lifeworld. It is always present, even if we are not aware of it at the moment. It is there whether or not we take notice of it.

Intentionality and meaning

The human existence, and consequently the lifeworld, is characterized by intentionality. In order to explicate lifeworld phenomenology we shall therefore make some acquaintance with this theory of phenomenology.

We often talk about intentions in the everyday language, for example that, 'my intention is to write a rich text'. However, the phenomenological idea of intentionality has little to do with this everyday use of the term, but concerns deeper dimensions of our lifeworld. Intentionality characterizes the most basic mode of being and refers to the relationship between a person and some object or event of her/his experience, or more simply, one's directed awareness of something in one's world (Husserl 1973/1948, 1998/1913, 2000/1928, Merleau-Ponty 1995/1945).

There is always an intentional relationship with the things that make up our everyday lives. Whatever we experience, it is experienced 'as something', and something that has meaning for us (also discussed by Smythe in Chapter 3). We experience the things that we use and that we see around us as the things, activity and places that belong to and signify our world. Even when we encounter an unfamiliar object, intentionality is active and helps us understand the object, at least as an 'unknown thing'.

It is because of our 'belongingness' to the world that we experience that things are always meaningful to us. Through this they bear explicit as well as implicit meaning that can be illuminated and clarified. Gadamer (1995/1960) expresses the idea:

> The intention and fulfilment of meaning belongs essentially to the unity of meaning, and like the meaning of the words that we use, every existing thing that has validity for me possesses correlatively and by virtue of its nature an 'ideal universality of actual and potential experiencing modes of givenness'.
>
> (Gadamer 1995/1960, p. 244)

Merleau-Ponty identifies that 'because we are in the world, we are condemned to meaning', (1995/1945, p. xix). Being in the world means that we cannot avoid meaning. Further, with a phenomenological approach professional carers and researchers are continuously searching for and encountering meaning, and are making efforts to describe these meanings in a clear and comprehensible way.

Even if intentionality and meaning are constantly there, in the lifeworld, in the daily life, it is not that easy to fully understand its on-going activity. In the moment of perceiving we tacitly experience the world in an all-at-once way, implicitly understanding what it means. When I sit down at my computer I never think that 'in order to key-in text I must first sit myself on the office chair, and lift my hands in the right level for the fingers to touch the keyboard'. I just sit down and start keying in text.

Intentionality and meaning is connected with context. When we see an object, such as a chair, its meaning is related to its spatial and temporal contexts. For example, a dinner table chair and an office chair could be very different, even if both essentially are chairs meant for comfortable sitting. Also the temporal aspects of the lifeworld are important. The characteristics of an object, again, such as a chair, differ with history; both in a general way and considering one's personal history. Even more important is the understanding of the relationship between, past, present and future. Sometimes the temporal aspects are understood as successive, that the present follows the past and moves into the future. However, the phenomenological understanding is that past, present and future are intertwined, and that every 'now' includes both present and future. In that perspective, 'now' is a nexus which connects the temporal horizons of the lifeworld. This means that we draw on all of our experience, both past and anticipated. Such experience becomes a moment in the present as we consider meanings and import for understanding and, for example, to make decisions.

Intentionality works silently and connects both spatial and temporal meanings. If writing academic texts earlier has been hard to me, I am likely to feel anguish when sitting down at my computer. If a previous childbirth has been a horrible experience, coming closer to the birthplace could make one feel bad, as it could harbour new unpleasant experiences. One problem is that all the aspects of the problematic experience are not immediately available. The negative feeling is sometimes just there, in a subtle way. It can be obvious and at the same time vague. It is not that the experiences are hard to grasp because they are 'forgotten', they dwell in intentionality. In that way they are as real as any manifest thing in the world.

Understanding intentionality in this way, we can see how meaning never is, and never can be, finally complete; there is thus no end to meaning. Meaning is infinite, always contextual, and recognized as expandable and expanding (Merleau-Ponty 1968/1948, 1995/1945). Consequently, meanings can be completed long after an event that once gave rise to them. With a sensitive approach, the intentional meanings can be made visible and in that way they can also change. The power of reworking meanings is limited only by our readiness to enlarge our experiences and understanding.

In a phenomenological approach to health care and research, intentionality and meaning are understood as situated in the human body as 'lived', and therefore the 'lived body' has an essential position here. Consequently, we must look closer at this central idea of lifeworld phenomenology.

The lived body

Merleau-Ponty (1995/1945) describes how we have access to a world through our bodies.[2] The idea of the lived body is essential to phenomenology, in which the human body never can be understood merely as a biological thing or as an object that can be moved around the room in the same way as furniture and other things. The body as a 'subjective object' is distinguishable from other objects in that we can turn away from the latter, whereas we can never turn away from the body. Instead, the body is constantly perceived and constantly perceiving. It is through the body and the bodily experience that the surrounding world becomes meaningful for us. 'My body is that meaningful core which behaves like a general function' as observed by Merleau-Ponty (p. 147). It is also the body that gives us a world in the first place, as it is 'our means of communication with it' (p. 92). It is the living body which offers a connection to the world and which carries out all living actions. 'The body is the vehicle of being in the world' (p. 82), 'our anchorage' (p. 144) in this world, and it is 'the horizon latent in all our experience and itself ever-present and anterior to every determining thought' (p. 92). We can never free ourselves from this embodiment, never come away from or stand outside of ourselves as lived bodies. As long as we live we have a world and the reason for that is the fact that we have a body. Or, as Merleau-Ponty emphasizes: a person does not 'have' a body, but 'is' her/his body.

According to phenomenological philosophy, human beings and their existence can never be understood without being considered as lifeworlds, as intentional and lived bodies. Measurements such as blood test results, scores, X-ray pictures and other so-called objective signs are important tools in health care, but are of limited value. Understanding a living person and her/his existence can never be complete without the perspective of her/his lived experience, her/his lived viewpoint of body, health, suffering and well-being.

Lifeworld phenomenology for caring

Essential to a lifeworld phenomenology for caring is the notion of health. In a new theory on health and caring (Dahlberg *et al.* 2009, Dahlberg and Segesten 2010) health is described in terms of well-being and a quality of 'being able to'. Health is thus more than biological health and freedom from disease. In a health care science approach, health means to feel well. Well-being is possible even if one is living with illness. Well-being is intertwined with the experience of existential vitality, having the power, lust and mood to carry through one's major as well as minor life projects. One such project is, of course, to bear and give birth to a child. Health and well-being also includes 'life rhythm', that one's life situation includes both 'movement' and 'stillness', where one side is not too dominant over the other. The sense of health, well-being and vitality can be strengthened by childbearing, birthing and motherhood, in which one fulfils a major life goal. However, such events can also be experienced as obstacles to a person's life projects. Whatever the circumstances, the woman's experiences of vitality, including life power, life lust, life mood and life rhythm must always be supported and strengthened, if the goal of care is health and well-being of mother and baby, as Berg and Lundgren (Lundgren 2004, Berg 2005, Lundgren and Berg 2007) as well as others have convincingly demonstrated.

'Health is silent', is an old saying. Gadamer (1996/1993) confirms this when he states that '[h]ealth does not actually present itself to us' (p. 107). There is a hidden character to health. When in health or well-being, one has an unreflected attitude to one's lived body and to the idea of health itself, which is taken for granted. This may be one explanation to why we talk so little of health within health care systems. Another explanation is the dominance of medicine and its focus on disease. However, in care that relates to childbearing and birthing, which most often is not about disease treatment, health care science has an important role to play, especially if it is inspired by lifeworld phenomenology and includes well-being, existential vitality and the quality of 'being able to'.

If the care of childbearing and birthing women (and possible partners) and their babies is to support and strengthen these persons' health, there must be some kind of lifeworld approach. This fundamental event of life when a new person is (to be) born has characteristics that are common to many, or even most, persons. There are, however, many aspects of the event that are strictly personal. There are experiences, and nuances of them, that are closely connected with everyone's own lifeworld, with one's own present situation, history and future of both temporal and spatial contexts. Especially now, when medicine and technology have provided this area of care with new settings and new expectations, which together with social and demographic changes create many questions that cannot be answered by one's own or other experienced mothers (or fathers), women need lifeworld sensitive care. A woman who is treated as an 'object', who does not feel seen or met, is likely to be less well prepared for birth and motherhood. With a lifeworld approach the right form of support can be given, the right 'presence' and 'hands-on comfort', which much research demonstrates the value of, can be offered (Berg 2005). We also know that support during childbirth increases breast-feeding rates, has a positive impact on mother–child bonding, and leads to fewer interventions (Hodnett *et al.* 2007). A lifeworld approach is a sound foundation for such support.

Here is where also the notion of lived body plays an important role. In a lifeworld approach, the lived body can be understood as a lifeworld communicator, which both conveys and absorbs existential meanings. In particular, the theory of the lived body illuminates the experiences of pain. Lundgren and Dahlberg (1998) and Nilsson and Lundgren (2009) have focused on fear of childbirth and how caring supports women (also discussed by Lundgren in Chapter 7). These authors describe how strong emotions come to play, even long before birthing is expected, and not least with women who host painful experiences from previous births. The pain and the experiences are not well understood by being reduced to 'memories' or 'cognitions', or even 'feelings'. Instead, painful experiences are more than that; they can dominate one's lifeworld and radically affect one's approach to the new childbearing period, the birthing as well as motherhood.

If, as Merleau-Ponty suggests, one is one's body, which in turn is one's access to life and also colours one's experience of life, a woman with these past experiences might have a very painful access to life. Her whole body lives that painful experience, as much 'here and now' as it did earlier. This also explains why a woman with a fear of childbirth can perceive her situation as being imprisoned – she is trapped by her (lived) body (Nilsson and Lundgren 2009). As a consequence, her self-image and self-esteem change, and she might be less able to become a mother. To adequately support these women they must be met as persons with dynamic lifeworlds and as lived bodies.

Sometimes childbearing, birthing and motherhood are affected by illness. When ill, (the loss of) health becomes clear and one does not enjoy easy and natural access to the world. Gadamer (1996/1993) states that illness is 'the loss of one's undisturbed "freedom"' and that it is a state that 'always involves a sort of exclusion from "life"' (p. 55). In illness, one is no longer free to participate in everyday activities or to fulfil one's goals and wishes of life. Illness is thus far more than symptoms, diagnoses, and treatment. It is the loss of abilities and the interruption of harmonic, easy and unmindful living. Illness makes clear what it means to have access to the world. When one's body is healthy and strong one meets the world unafraid. When one is ill, one's body becomes an obstacle that keeps one from immediate engagement and it alters one's attachment with the world. Toombs (1993) purports that a break down of one's body means a break down of life.

The meaning of health and illness that is connected with childbearing, birthing and motherhood is particularly profound. There is an extra dimension to the care that should support and strengthen the experience of health as well-being, existential vitality and the experience of 'being able to'. Consequently, lifeworld phenomenology, including the notions of lived body, is also profound. Grounded in the lifeworld, professional carers, including nurses and midwives, can support well-being even if illness dominates the situation, and support the person's power to go through with the events that give life to a new person, as well as to a new life project, filled with a myriad of meanings.

Lifeworld phenomenology for health care research

Phenomenology does not only provide us with insights into health and caring, but is a rich source for researchers to find ways to illuminate human existence in the context of caring. The lifeworld theory, together with the notions of intentionality and 'lived body', offers methodological tools with which the multilayered world of humanity is revealed and understood. The overall aim of lifeworld research is the description and elucidation of the lived world in a way that expands our understanding of human experience, including health and well-being. With phenomenology it becomes possible to confront the human everyday world in a scientific way that clarifies the lifeworld underpinnings of any explanations that science might propose.

However, research with lifeworld phenomenology as a foundation must often be defended for not dealing with mathematics and, consequently, for not being scientific enough. Therefore we must begin the methodological discussion with a consideration of the use of numbers.

My son works with financial analyses. Depending on his calculations, big money transactions are made. I once asked him if he ever runs into the problem of immeasurable phenomena in his analyses. 'Yes, of course I do', he replied. I then asked him how he behaves when this happens. He looked a bit puzzled but said, 'I describe them, the texts in my reports are as impor-tant as the tables of figures'. I pushed a bit saying, 'You do not put numbers on them then?' 'Of course not', he said, 'I cannot put numbers on things that are not measurable'. When I told him that this is exactly what happens in health care research, his spontaneous answer was, that 'well, that's weak science then'.

It is indeed unscientific to force immeasurable phenomena into matrices that reduce them to measurable entities, sometimes beyond our ability to recognize them. And we do not have to. Both pre-dating and parallel to the on-going scientific movement there are approaches to science and research which are based in words, stories and texts. Besides the treasure of European continental philosophy, there is a long and world-wide movement of phe-nomenology, as is shown by Tymieniecka (2002) in an extensive anthology. This philosophy is a rich well that can nourish health care researchers who want to scientifically explore and describe health related issues. There is obviously no need to despair in a false lack of scientific methodology when the phenomena in focus do not match mathematics.

Phenomenology begins within and deals with the lifeworld. As noted above it was Husserl's contention that science begins with and extends from a lifeworld perspective. As a matter of fact, all science and all researchers are in the lifeworld realm. Even scientists are human beings who, like all others, live and work within and through a lifeworld. But unlike humans in general, Husserl (1973/1948, 1998/1913, 2000/1928) teaches us that, as scientists, we need to understand how the lifeworld helps as well as hinders us to describe what we experience and come to see through our research. We need to be aware of how the ever-existing lifeworld affects the results of our studies, and their quality. We thus need a phenomenological under-standing of methodology and the meaning of what is commonly described as the characteristics of science: validity, objectivity and generalisability.[3]

Phenomenology methodology

Phenomenology offers a key to an explicit and reflective grounding of science in the lifeworld (an approach that later was adopted by hermeneu-tics). The phenomenological concept of the lifeworld implies ontology as well as epistemology and methodology for health science research in which the question of meaning is primary. Health science phenomenology seeks to understand the meanings of health related phenomena in our everyday experiences of health, well-being and illness. These meanings are often implicit, 'tacit' and taken for granted and it is through the research that the implied meaning becomes explicit, can be seen and heard, problematized and reflected upon.

On the way from implicit meanings to explicit descriptions we move from unique experiences to descriptions that are valid to persons other than those involved in our research. To work with this is a delicate matter. Researchers must in the first place know how to catch the lifeworld meanings, all the exemplars and nuances. Without losing the richness, one must then find a way to describe the outcome of one's scientific endeavour.

In the following, I will give my view of how lifeworld phenomenology serves the scientific purposes of research, and describe a phenomenological way of looking at what is commonly described as 'data collection'and 'data analysis'. Before entering the research handicraft we shall take a deeper look at the research approach, the attitude and tone that must characterize all phenomenological research, the design of the study as well as its presentation, and both data collection and data analysis. First however we shall explore how an idea of 'bridling' can help us not to get lost when we try to find our way through the lifeworld exhibitions.

The need for bridling

Referring to Husserl, Gadamer (1995/1960) asserts that the lifeworld itself is tacit. It is 'the world in which we are immersed in the "natural" and unreflective attitude that never becomes an object as such for us, but that represents the pre-given basis of all experience' (pp. 246–247). Like Gadamer, Merleau-Ponty emphasizes our immediate and silent anchorage in the world. He wants us to carefully investigate the bonds to the world and the complexity of understanding the world as well as the pre-understanding that makes up the lifeworld. He began his 'Causeries' on French radio and broadcast 1948 with the words:

> The world of perception, or in other words the world which is revealed to us by our senses and in everyday life, seems at first sight to be the one we know best of all. For we need neither to measure nor to calculate in order to gain access to this world and it would seem that we can fathom it simply by opening our eyes and getting on with our lives. Yet this is a delusion. In these lectures I hope to show that the world of perception is, to a great extent, unknown territory as long as we remain in the practical or utilitarian attitude.
>
> (Merleau-Ponty 2004/1948, p. 39)

The lifeworld is consequently something that is pre-given and implicit for science and scientifically based praxis. At the same time as our experience of engagement is an indispensable prerequisite of our existence, it poses an epistemological problem. We cannot completely rely on perception. We know from our everyday experience how we often see things that are not really there. We also do not see things that are there, ready for perception to be grasped, but which are overseen by us. A foundational demand of researchers in the service of science is to be able to examine the acts of intentionality, to see when and how meanings come to be. As researchers we need to go beyond the natural attitude of everyday experience in favour of a reflective stance. We need 'bridling' (Dahlberg *et al.* 2008).[4]

Researchers must practise a disciplined kind of interaction and communication with phenomena and informants, and 'bridle' the event of understanding so that we do not understand too quickly, too carelessly or in a slovenly manner. Instead of a quick decision of what something *is* or what meaning is being discovered, as researchers we must systematically and carefully scrutinize the road to the decision of understanding. 'Bridling' means an open, respectful, sensitive and alert attitude of actively waiting for the phenomenon to show up and display itself within the relationship, with the researcher taking the role of a hunter of meanings. The aim of 'bridling' is to slow the evolving understanding in order to more clearly see the phenomenon – its nuances as well as its essentials.

Researchers practise phenomenology in order to understand the meaning of lifeworld phenomena (see also Chapters 7 and 9 for examples of research which have utilized a lifeworld phenomenological approach). Describing meanings includes clarification of meanings that are explicitly grasped as well as those more hidden, inferred or implicit meanings that also belong to all phenomena. Accordingly, researchers should be aware that the meanings that are discovered belong to the phenomena in focus, and should avoid supplying the understanding with meanings that do not belong there. In research, one must pay attention to how, in what way, phenomena are being illuminated and how, in what way their meanings are made explicit. Consequently, 'bridling' is the main phenomenological answer to questions of validity and objectivity. It is the scientific attitude that must be activated through all the research; in the planning, in the phase of data collection, in the analysis, as well as in the presentation of research results. There is no scientific procedure that can save validity or objectivity if 'bridling' is not being practised.

Getting in touch with people's lifeworlds

In health care research, including the research of childbearing and birthing, we want to know how everything in this field is to the people involved, in particular to the mothers, fathers and babies. What meaning is there in childbearing, to the mother to be, the father to be? What does birthing mean to the mother, to the father? What is the meaning of pain? What is the meaning of joy and how is it supported? What is the meaning of life lust or life mood when a new life is entering the stage of existence? What is the meaning of breast-feeding to the mother, to the father, or to the baby? In order to understand the meaning of these things we have to be able to understand the people involved, we have to get access to their lifeworlds.

The language of the lifeworld is prose (Merleau-Ponty 1991/1969, 1995/1945). When we in everyday life want a fellow human being to understand something we simply tell her/him a short or longer story about that thing. If necessary, we include details, nuances and perhaps metaphors in order for the message to be clear and understandable. This everyday ability is what we build upon even in research, and we ask our 'informants' to describe a phenomenon and its meanings to us, orally in an interview, or written as a narrative, for example, in a diary. However, in research we are aware of the multifaceted lifeworld, the multilayered intentionality and the many tacit meanings that are there, and that researchers have to be more careful with understanding. This is an example of where 'bridling' is important. When we get a description, such as 'That was a wonderful midwife', we have to ask, 'How do you mean?', 'Wonderful, in what way?', 'Can you tell me more about that?' In order not to take for granted what particular descriptions mean, follow-up questions must be posed. In general, researchers use all too few of these questions or invitations to tell more, to give more descriptions in detail, to present more lifeworld variants.

Sometimes, however, talking is not appropriate. If we want to understand something in the lifeworld of babies, we cannot practise interviews. Even with adults, interviewing can fall short: for example, if they cannot speak at all, or if there are experiences that are deeply embedded or otherwise problematic to talk about. To use 'observation' as a means to get research data is one way to come closer to embodied experiences that are hard to capture, as well as hard to verbalize. As researchers, we can also use whatever means of everyday life that help us understand something, for example drawings, paintings, and poems (Dahlberg 2006a).

In one way or another, whatever means we use in a study, it must be transformed into verbal language, at least in the reporting of the research. Using observation and similar data sources clearly raises a problem. In interviewing, it is the informants who give words to the experiences. Using methods such as observation, it is we, the researchers, who give words to the experience. This is unavoidable. However, in the light of phenomenological philosophy, which is confirmed by my lived experience from years of research, I propose that all types of data collection, such as observations and the use of drawings, should be complemented by interviewing or other kinds of dialogues, if possible. The point is that, in order not to take too much for granted, we need the phenomenon to be expressed by the people involved.[5]

Describing structures of meaning

Once the lifeworld descriptions have been obtained the analysis of meaning can begin. The data descriptions must be 'rich' in order for structures and essences to be found. This means that they should include many aspects of the phenomenon. In other words, there should be a wealth of variations of the phenomenon. The goal is to understand that structure of meaning that describes a phenomenon of interest, preferably in a new way, teaching us something new about the phenomenon (Dahlberg 2006b).

In the attitude of 'bridling', researchers carry on the analysis by questioning data about what is being said about the phenomenon in focus, how it is said and what the meaning is. How does the interviewee describe the phenomenon? What does s/he really say? Is a particular comment really an expression of an understanding of the focused phenomenon or is another object in focus? How do the different utterances fit with each other within the framework of a single person's narrative? Does the interviewee express more than one understanding? If so, do they agree with one another? Are there also opposing statements or observations? What do such controversies mean? Is something continually repeated? What do the descriptions evoke in me as researcher? What do I recognize? What is surprising to me? What do I think? What do I feel?

The phenomenological analysis is characterized by a search for the meanings that are explicitly or implicitly conveyed by the descriptions in data. To illuminate hidden meanings, one sometimes has to work hard with the data. One way to discover meanings and to see structures of meanings is to make clusters of meaning, which is an important intermediate stage on the way to a final description. At the same time, this phase of the analysis should not be over emphasized. The clusters are not part of the findings and are not seen in the presentation of the findings. The clusters are more a framework for a temporary pattern of meanings that helps the researcher to see structures of meanings that describe and explicate the phenomenon, its characteristic features, its essence.

'Phenomenology is the study of essences', Merleau-Ponty (1995/1945, p. vii) reports in his previously mentioned famous preface to *Phenomenology of Perception*. Essences belong to the world that is 'already there'; they belong 'already' to the lifeworld and the everyday manner of which we live our lives. Consequently, essences are not something that we as researchers explicitly add to the research. Essences are not produced or constructed by us. They are there already, in the intentional relationship between the phenomena and us. Merleau-Ponty states:

> [We cannot] conceive the perceiving subject as a consciousness which 'interprets', 'deciphers', or 'orders' a sensible matter according to an ideal law which it possesses. Matter is 'pregnant' with its form ...
>
> (Merleau-Ponty 1964/1946, p. 12)

Essences belong to the in-between world, that 'single fabric' that connects us with everything else in the world, with other subjects or objects. As Merleau-Ponty (1968/1948) posited, essences belong to the 'flesh of the world'.

Researchers who aim to describe structures of meaning and essences can never follow a method as one follows a path that has been staked out beforehand. The process of analysis is characterized by a balance between free discovery and attachment to certain scientific guidelines, such as 'bridling'. Researchers within phenomenology must learn how to patiently wait to see something to hang on to. They need to be able to tolerate uncertainty and the 'woolly' or awkward feelings that follow when one does not know exactly what is going on and what the result will be. This kind of research requires the formulation of questions at the outset of the research, but it also requires the reformulation of old questions and the discovery of new ones as each study unfolds.[6]

The concrete work of the analysis is best understood in terms of 'figure and background'. First of all, the essence as a figure can be seen to stand out against its background, the particulars, the nuances and variations of the phenomenon. Further, to work in terms of 'figure and background' means to 'play' with the different meanings that are present in data. The attention is directed towards discovering a pattern of meanings, a pattern of clusters of meaning. However, when 'wading about' in the multitude of meanings it is important to work actively with the emerging meanings: picking up one meaning and watching it as a figure against the others as background, then picking up another cluster of meaning and making it a temporary figure, and so on. One moment an explicit tentative meaning is a figure, the next the same part of the text and its meaning is part of the background. In this event of movement there is sooner or later stillness. Some relationships of meanings become obvious and in such way the essential structure of meanings can be conveyed.

However, all structures of meaning, or essences, are open, infinite and expandable and they are never completely explored and described. Meaning emerges in relation to 'events' of the lifeworld, and when the lifeworld changes, meaning changes as well. To make the whole structure of meaning explicit is important, as it covers the most essential parts as well as the more manifest and contextual events of the phenomenon in focus. That way, it is possible for the reader to judge how far and in what way a research result can be transferred to other situations and contexts than the original.

There is always the risk that essences are separated from existence by language (Merleau-Ponty 1995/1945). It can be tempting to arrive at high theoretical levels with the analysis. Researchers might want to create theories from their research. This is possible, but researchers must be open and sensitive to the original lifeworld descriptions, the phenomenon and its open horizons.

Preferably, a phenomenological account is 'phenomenon oriented', meaning that it is focused on the essence of the phenomenon. However, results are often 'person oriented', or focused on the idiographic. 'There is a big risk if we are captivated by the various individual experiences which are reported, especially the hard or otherwise extreme ones; that is, we are too subject oriented' (Hallberg *et al.* 2010). A move from the variations of personal experiences to the essential features of the phenomenon, therefore becoming phenomenon oriented, does not demand that the researcher leaves the personal and contextual meanings behind. The opposite is the case. The moral concern for and the interest of the person is still valid. Even in enquiry aimed at the essence of phenomena it is the obligation of the researcher to illuminate the variations that are the foundation of the meaning structure. The obligation of phenomenology is always the illumination of the lifeworld. It begins in the lifeworld and ends in the lifeworld.

Conclusion

Lifeworld phenomenology is a rich source for practitioners and researchers in the health care area who want to illuminate and better understand phenomena and their meanings related to childbearing and birthing. The phenomenological enterprise is to a great extent a matter of balancing and intertwining existential aspects, which sometimes seem to be opposites or poles apart in dichotomies. Within a phenomenological approach, health care practitioners and researchers must be able to embrace complexities, even ambiguities. Lifeworld phenomenology offers scientific answers that allows for meanings of health to be revealed in the midst of illness and for unique lived experiences to be included in essences. In the phenomenological realm, theory is not apart from practise, but intertwined with it.

Notes

1 I have studied especially 1900's European philosophy, in particular the continental tradition, with the purpose of outlining an epistemological foundation for methodological work. While working on this I found that the philosophy could not only serve the epistemological and methodological needs of human science in general but caring science in particular. Especially the German and French philosophy that is called phenomenology (sometimes, existential philosophy) which describes the human existence in such a way that it also addresses the questions that we have in the field of health care.
Epistemological and methodological results of the empirical and the philosophical analyses have been published in several articles, and synthesized in a book: Dahlberg K., Dahlberg H. and Nyström M. (2008) *Reflective Lifeworld Research* (2nd rev. edn), Studentlitteratur: Lund. Another synthesis resulted in a book on health and caring: Dahlberg K. and Segesten K. (2010) *Hälsa och vårdande – i teori och praxis (Health and Caring – in theory and praxis)*. Stockholm: Natur & Kultur. Some parts of this article originate from these monographs.
2 It is nevertheless wrong to say that Merleau-Ponty's philosophy is mainly characterized by his idea of the lived body, or that it is anthropology. Rather, Merleau-Ponty's philosophy is best characterized as an ontology, i.e. a philosophy of 'the flesh of the world' (cf. 1968).

3 Cf. Husserl (2000/1928). See also Dahlberg *et al.* (2008).
4 The idea of 'bridling' is published in Dahlberg (2006b) and Dahlberg *et al.* (2008). I prefer the term 'bridling' before the more common term 'bracketing', because 'bridling' is directed forwards at the whole event of understanding. 'Bracketing' is directed backwards, putting all energy into fighting pre-understanding and keeping it in check 'back there'.
5 Cf. Dahlberg (2006a,b). If the informants are babies who cannot be dialogued in any way, one must try to involve other sources, e.g. other studies, parents, professional carers, etc.
6 Cf. the chapter on openness in Dahlberg *et al.* (2008).

References

Berg M. (2005). A midwifery model of care for childbearing women at high risk: genuine caring in caring for the genuine. *Journal of Perinatal Education* 14, (1), 9–21.

Dahlberg K. (2006a). 'The individual in the world – the world in the individual': towards a human science phenomenology that includes the social world. *Indo-Pacific Journal of Phenomenology* 6 August (www.jpip.org).

Dahlberg K. (2006b). The essence of essences – the search for meaning structures in phenomenological analysis of lifeworld phenomena. *International Journal of Qualitative Studies on Health and Well-being* 1 (1), 11–19.

Dahlberg K., Berg M. and Lundgren I. (1999). Commentary. Studying maternal experiences of childbirth. *Birth* 29 (4), 215–217.

Dahlberg K., Dahlberg H. and Nyström M. (2008). *Reflective Lifeworld Research* (2nd. rev. edn). Studentlitteratur: Lund.

Dahlberg K., Todres L. and Galvin K. (2009). Lifeworld-led healthcare is more than patient-led care: an existential view of well-being. *Medicine, Health Care and Philosophy* 12 (3), 265–271.

Dahlberg K. and Segesten K. (2010). *Hälsa och vårdande – I teori och praxis* (*Health and caring – in theory and praxis*). Natur & Kultur: Stockholm.

Gadamer H-G. (1995/1960). *Truth and Method.* (2nd rev. Edn) (J. Weinsheimer and D. Marshall, trans.). The Continuum Publishing Company: New York.

Gadamer H-G. (1996/1993). *The Enigma of Health* (J. Gaiger and N. Walker, trans.). Stanford University Press: Stanford, CA.

Hallberg L., Dahlberg K. and Ashworth P.D. (2010). Editorial. *International Journal of Qualitative Studies on Health and Well-being* 5 (1). DOI: 10.3402/qhw.v5i1.4987.

Hodnett E.D., Gates S., Hofmeyr G.J. and Sakala C. (2007). Continuous support for women during childbirth. *Cochrane Database of Systematic Reviews* (3), CD003766.

Husserl E. (1970/1936). *The Crisis of European Sciences and Transcendental Phenomenology* (D. Carr, trans.). North Western University Press: Evanston, IL.

Husserl E. (1973/1948). *Experience and Judgement* (J.S. Churchill and K. Ameriks, trans.). North Western University Press: Evanston, IL.

Husserl E. (1998/1913). *Ideas Pertaining to a Pure Phenomenology and to a Phenomenological Philosophy. First Book* (F. Kersten, trans.). Kluwer Academic Publication: Dordrecht.

Husserl E. (2000/1928). *Ideas Pertaining to a Pure Phenomenology and to a Phenomenological Philosophy. Second Book* (R. Rojcewicz and A. Schuwer, trans.). Kluwer Academic Publication: Dordrecht.

Lundgren I. (2004). Releasing and relieving encounters – experiences of pregnancy and childbirth. *Scandinavian Journal of Caring Sciences* 18, 368–375.

Lundgren I. and Dahlberg K. (1998). Women's experience of pain during childbirth. *International Journal of Midwifery* 14, 105–110.

Lundgren I. and Berg M. (2007). Central concept in the midwife–woman relationship. *Scandinavian Journal of Caring Sciences* 21, 220–228.

Merleau-Ponty M. (1964/1946). The primacy of perception and its philosophical consequences. In *The Primacy of Perception* (J. Edie, trans.). North Western University Press: Evanston, IL.

Merleau-Ponty M. (1968/1948). *The Visible and the Invisible* (A. Lingis, trans). North Western University Press: Evanston, IL.

Merleau-Ponty M. (1991/1969). *The Prose of the World* (J. O'Neill, trans.). North Western University Press: Evanston, IL.

Merleau-Ponty M. (1995/1945). *Phenomenology of Perception* (C. Smith, trans.). Routledge: London.

Merleau-Ponty M. (2004/1948). *The World of Perception* (O. Davies, trans.). Routledge: London.

Nilsson C. and Lundgren I. (2009). Women's lived experience of fear of childbirth. *International Journal of Midwifery* 25, 1–9.

Toombs K. (1993). *The Meaning of Illness: A Phenomenological Account of the Different Perspectives of Physician and Patient*. Kluwer Academic Publishers: Boston.

Tymieniecka M-T. (2002). *Phenomenology Worldwide. Foundations – Expanding Dynamics – Life-Engagements. A Guide for Research and Study*. Kluwer Academic Publishers: Dordrecht.

3 From beginning to end

How to do hermeneutic interpretive phenomenology

Elizabeth Smythe

Introduction

This chapter is written specifically to assist a person to do hermeneutic interpretive phenomenology. I write it in a similar manner to that which I take thesis students through their lived experience of such a journey. Thus, I present advice in the same order as I believe 'works' in enacting this methodological approach. The suggestions are equally relevant for any research report using this methodological approach. Heidegger (1889–1976) and Gadamer (1900–2002) are the two key philosophers who inform hermeneutic interpretive phenomenology and whose philosophical notions are inherent in the statements above. Insights from their writing will be addressed throughout the chapter at points when one needs to link understanding with action. An overview of the hermeneutic interpretive phenomenological process is also depicted in Figure 3.1 on page 52.

The phenomenological world of practice

I remember the day so clearly. I was a very new midwife working in delivery suite. It was busy. The woman I was with began to push. I rang the bell for help. A young medical student came; to observe. The baby came swiftly and was born flat and floppy. As we turned our attention to the baby at the same time I realised this woman was bleeding more than normal. I rang the bell again, twice. The bleeding got worse. I rang the three emergency bells, long and persistent. Still nobody came. Meanwhile the baby had come around, but the bleeding was a nightmare. As I rushed around to draw up ecbolics I realised the floor was awash with blood and liquor; another danger. This was not how the textbooks described a post-partum haemorrhage (PPH). When one rings for help, help comes. They do not tell you about the flat baby and the PPH happening at the same time, nor the slippery floor that makes movement treacherous. They do not even hint that another woman in the delivery unit could be having a cardiac arrest at the same time as the junior midwife has her first emergency. They do not explain how to keep calm amidst feelings of panic. Maternal mortality statistics bear no resemblance to the experience of seeing a woman's life blood pour forth relentlessly. Textbooks do not colour practice with the hues that show in experience itself.

(Author)

Experience is how life 'is'. Midwifery practice, as described above in my account of 30 years ago, is always amidst a context that offers possibilities and/or creates havoc. Theoretical knowledge in itself is not sufficient to equip one to know what to do: situations are always unique. One may be thrown into the midst of having to respond beyond one's experience or capabilities. Who 'is' or 'is not' there makes a difference. How one's heart thumps has an impact; time can rush by or hang in slowness. Responsibility weighs heavy in one's heart. Thinking becomes embodied as one simply reacts, drawing on the thoughts that come, trying this and trying that; always watching; always anticipating what could happen next; trying to get on top of the danger. Midwifery practice (as part of life itself) is in the midst of a situation where anything can happen, at any time. One can call oneself 'competent' but in the moment of slipping on a wet floor undermine that completely. At the same time, we are in the midst of the ever-evolving physiological processes of mother and baby. The situation is always dynamic. What is still to come is always unknown. Such is the phenomenological world of practice.

Assumptions of the hermeneutic interpretive paradigm

Knowing the lived nature of each practice encounter draws me again and again to hermeneutic interpretive phenomenology. This research approach is based on the following.

- Understanding is deeply informed by experience.
- Such lived-understanding is often covered over, taken for granted and/or silenced amidst theoretical/scientific discourse.
- Each situation is unique, dynamic and informed by what has been and influenced by what is still to come.
- Every situation is in a context, where people, place, time, mood, resources, rules, global events, local gossip, a rainy day, untold influences come together.
- Within the uniqueness of human experience there is understanding that resonates with others.
- Truth is covered over; hidden. The quest is to come nearer to understanding; to think. Truth as the whole truth always remains elusive.
- In telling a story, experience begins its interpretive journey. One can never replicate experience 'as it was', as one only ever talks of particular aspects from a certain perspective. Meaning lies between the lines of what is said, to be uncovered.

- A researcher can only offer his or her interpretation of another's story for the purpose of raising questions, pondering, offering pointers to understanding. The interpretation does not claim to state 'what was meant', but rather to open a conversation with readers as to possible understandings. Findings are tentative, suggestive, possibilities.
- Researchers cannot free themselves from their own unique pre-understandings which will always bias their thinking. Language itself is used by the researcher in a way that already holds prejudice. The challenge is for the researcher to seek to become aware of the nature of their prejudices and alert the reader to how they may influence the study. Further, the research seeks to be open to hearing and thinking beyond 'already there' understandings.
- The quest is to provide a research report that enables the audience to engage with experience as lived by others, to ponder afresh the phenomenon in question, and to be taken-along on a showing, thinking pathway which invites more questions.

Choosing the methodology

Many people will tell you to first decide on your research question and then identify the most fitting methodology. I confess that my doctoral research began with my decision that I wanted to use phenomenology. I chose the methodology first. My later experience of supervising research students is that some really struggle with the free flowing, let-the-thoughts come nature of phenomenology. I believe some people are naturally attuned to phenomenology, while others are not. Consider the following questions.

- Do you respond more to the opportunity to be creative rather than to follow a clear set of rules?
- Are you drawn to beautiful writing, to poetry?
- Can you hear what lies behind what people say?
- Do you tend to do more listening than talking?
- If you are walking, driving or in some other solitary activity do you find yourself lost in thought?
- Can you read philosophy without necessarily understanding, but keep on reading because you sense that understanding might come?
- Do you enjoy writing in a manner in which you get lost in the writing; the words just flow?
- Is there something about the nature of 'being human' that intrigues and delights you?
- Are you drawn to tell affirming stories?
- Can you 'trust the process'? That is, continue on without being sure of where you are going but trusting that you somehow know the way?

- Would you be content to finish your study in the humility of knowing there is still much you do not yet understand?
- When your findings resonate, and you get the phenomenological nod of 'Yes, that's how it is', are you comfortable knowing you have uncovered what people already knew but perhaps had forgotten, or had never quite put into words before?

If you find yourself nodding to most of these questions, then read on. If not, then you may need to find a more structured research approach, or one that addresses power issues more explicitly, or one that comes up with findings that offer a stronger sense of 'truth', or one that deals specifically with the question that interests you.

There is one issue you need to consider before you settle on your decision to draw on the writing of Heidegger. That is, the question of Heidegger's association with the Nazi party (Lang 1996, Young 1997, Collins 2000, Harman 2007) (also discussed by Healy in Chapter 12). My own stance is that he was influenced by the context of the times, and his later silence on the atrocities is open to multiple interpretations. The critique seems to lie with his behaviour, not with any fascist qualities within his writing. Asking such questions keeps the researcher mindful of the danger of being held by unrecognized fascist assumptions.

The research question

The research question in the hermeneutic interpretive approach is very simple. There are five words that tend to feature: 'how', 'lived', 'experience', 'being', and 'meaning'. 'How' seeks to uncover 'the way' of something, how it 'is' in the living of it. That means, this approach does not ask 'why'; it does not problem solve, explain or seek to control. (Examples of research which have utilized a hermeneutic/interpretive phenomenological approach are presented in Chapters 5, 6, 8, 10 and 12). Van Manen's classic text *Researching Lived Experience* (1990), a guide I strongly recommend, brings the words 'lived' and 'experience' together, saying such an approach is to 'question the way we experience the world, to want to know the world in which we live as human beings' (p. 5). There are differing opinions on whether one needs to be explicit in talking of experience as 'lived', or whether the very nature of the word 'experience' always already relates back to what has been lived. Similarly, the word 'being' carries with it the notion that being is living experience. 'Meaning' takes us to the quest of seeking to understand; as opposed to describing, arguing, predicting, deconstructing, theorizing. The question for my doctoral study was 'what is the meaning of being safe in relation to childbirth?' (Smythe 1998, 2003). Equally, I could have worded the question as 'how is it to be safe in childbirth?' or 'what is the experience of being safe...?'

The phenomenon

At the heart of a phenomenological study is a phenomenon; that which 'shows itself in itself' (Heidegger 1995, p. 51). The phenomenon of my study was 'being safe'. The challenge Heidegger presents to us is that a phenomenon is never on show complete in itself. It lies hidden, needing uncovering. It can appear (for example when the midwife tells me about how she assesses the woman). It can be announced (the scan report announces). But the phenomenon can also show as seeming to be safe when it is not safe at all. That is the ever-present question of phenomenological research. A woman in my study told the story of her baby becoming very dehydrated. She had midwives who always seemed too busy to stop and help or even stop and listen. 'They asked the question "are the nappies wet?" but not "how wet?". I had no idea they were supposed to be that wet' (Smythe 1988, p. 196). Those midwives were enacting the semblance of being safe. How often does the semblance disguise negligent or disinterested care? Finding meaning is to play with the possibilities of semblance, the taken-for-granted, the assumed. It is to ask of every appearance, 'could this seem to be, but not be, the thing itself at all?'

Holding the focus

Naming the phenomenon of one's study is to place that as the keystone of thinking, questioning, listening, reading and writing. Everything becomes focused on the phenomenon. At the end of the study one presents a synthesis of writing that seeks to capture the nature of how participants experienced the phenomenon. While individual stories are vital to the 'showing', it is the phenomenon which rises to the fore. Amidst rich research data there is always danger of stories captivating interest that do not directly relate to the phenomenon of the question. Those stories are to be put aside. The discipline amidst the free-flowing nature of this approach is the researcher's unwavering commitment to the named phenomenon.

Ethics approval

My advice is to seek ethics approval early in your study so you can begin interviewing straight away. The data must lead a hermeneutic interpretive phenomenological study. The main ethical consideration is to recognize the impact of having someone listen to one's story. Phenomenology draws out everyday stories that people are not used to telling, and/or much longer stories than the quick version that crops up in conversation. Such story telling can bring participants to emotional vulnerability. It is very common for tears to be part of the phenomenological interview. When listened to in a supportive, empathic manner, participants report the value of such an opportunity. Nevertheless, the researcher needs to be mindful that they may open up memories that require follow-up professional counselling.

Pre-understandings

There is a waiting time during the ethical approval process. That is an ideal time for the research supervisor to interview the researcher on their own experience of the phenomenon. The purpose of this is to draw forth their own stories so they may become mindful of the assumptions and prejudices they carry with them into the study. Heidegger (1995) suggests we find it hardest to see that which is closest. It is by telling our own stories and then going back to review them as though they were from a participant that we begin to glimpse how values, past experience, vested interest, culture, role etc. shape the way we understand and experience the world.

The Heideggerian way

As outlined by Dowling in Chapter 4, the Heideggerian way is a key differentiation from a Husserlian approach. (Insights into Heidegger's philosophies and methodological application are also presented by Healy in Chapter 12.) Gadamer, following on from Heidegger's (1995) notion that we always approach phenomenon with fore-having (already there knowing), fore-sight (the ability to imagine how it might be) and fore-conception (the ideas we bring) says, 'The important thing is to be aware of one's own bias, so that the text may present itself in all its newness and thus be able to assert its own truth against one's own fore-meanings' (1982, p. 238). He nevertheless reminds us of the 'tyranny of hidden prejudices' (p. 239). Interpretation is always 'my own'. This became clear to me when a participant in my study told me how unsafe her midwife was because when she was in labour, all swollen up with pre-eclampsia, the midwife put a drip up to give her intravenous fluids. My participant had no understanding that this was 'safe practice'. She saw it as making her even more swollen. My midwifery lens gave me a different interpretation. I knew that fluid in the tissues leaves the woman with reduced fluid in her circulation. The crux of this story was not who was right and who was wrong, but rather revealed mis-interpretations in the practice encounter. It could be argued that as an interpreter with an understanding of the scientific knowledge base of practice, my interpretation in this instance had a 'legitimate prejudice' (Gadamer 1982, p. 246). Nevertheless, Gadamer suggests the quest of hermeneutics is to seek to 'recapture the perspective' (ibid., p. 259) from which this woman made her statement. In a situation of already feeling unsafe, when the midwife inserted the intravenous fluids the woman's understanding of what this meant made her feel even more unsafe. That is the issue. The interpretive lens of the researcher is one of courage, informed by all one's understandings drawn from life experience to make sense of the meaning inherent in the story. It was my background as a practising midwife that enabled my prejudices and helped me to see beyond what was said. I could not divorce myself from such understanding.

Method

How long since…?

Participants need to have had the experience. It depends on the impact of their experiences as to how fresh they will be in their memories. There is no right time from which to gain the perfect perspective. A woman's experience of birth is likely to be recounted in a different manner immediately after the baby is born, to the next day, the next week, or the next year. Years later the story will still be the same but again the perspective will have altered. When people asked about my PhD, women who had given birth decades earlier started telling me their stories with amazing clarity. The researcher simply needs to consider the point of perspective that is likely to have the most relevance, and be appropriate for the participants.

Who?

One seeks stories from participants; they therefore need to have stories to tell. It is helpful if there is a common language, and that the person is skilled in capturing the description and mood of what happened. While all will have experienced a common phenomenon, the researcher may choose to purposely select people with a variety of experiences. This is to spark thinking, not to make comparative statements about different categories.

How many?

The number of participants depends on the time available to conduct the research. My experience suggests that in a masters study (one year, full time) five to eight participants are likely to yield as much data as one can think through. For a doctoral study the number may increase to between 12 to 20 participants. There is certainly an upper limit. One seeks to honour each participant by working intensively with their data. The thinking that emerges from such analysis becomes embodied. One reaches a state of 'knowing' that one more interview will be too many. Already the insights are emerging like a river of thought. To keep pouring in more runs the risk of overflowing the banks which somehow hold the thoughts in a coherent whole.

How many interviews?

If the topic of the research is about distinct events, such as a woman's experience of labour, then I believe one interview is enough. A person tells their story and it is done. While it is good to have permission to go back to clarify details, a second interview is likely to feel redundant. On the other hand, if the participants are to talk of experiences that are so common they struggle to distinguish one from another, a series of interviews may help them to talk about 'yesterday' with descriptive clarity. For example, asking a midwife about her experience of conducting antenatal assessments may be difficult for her as she has done so many, but she can recall the most recent one she has done. The first interview may help her to be more attuned in her subsequent practice and thus enable her to tell stories with more clarity at a second interview.

The research conversation

The quest of hermeneutic interpretive phenomenology is to return as closely as possible to the primordial experience, that is, the un-worded 'being' (Heidegger 1995). To draw a participant into conversation is to encourage them to bring words to shape, colour and texture the account of what happened. To stay close to experience itself is to recount the story itself. Questions therefore need to prompt such telling: 'Tell me what happened?', 'And then what happened?', 'How did you feel?'. A person in story-telling mode is likely to continue with little need for on-going prompts.

Sometimes it is hard to elicit a story, especially when the experience is common. Useful prompts are: 'Tell me about the last time…', 'Tell be about a time that went really well…', 'Tell me about a challenging time…', 'Tell me about yesterday…'.

Fiumara (1990) reminds us that: 'The listening attitude …determines what the speaker will say as much as the speaker himself determines it' (p. 145). I cannot tell you how to listen; but I can tell you that you yourself will influence the openness of the participant.

The nature of human experience is that participants are likely to have already engaged in their own process of analysis. They may readily move into a more interpretive telling, drawn from generalized experience, offering opinions. While such data can still be accommodated under a more hermeneutic lens, I encourage a quest to stay focused on stories. Such data brings a much richer potential for analysis.

It is easy for both participant and researcher to get caught up in the story telling. I recommend two tape recorders for the all too common moments when attention is distracted and the recording goes awry.

If the researcher has time to transcribe the interviews themselves it is a useful way of becoming very familiar with the data in an attuned manner. Nevertheless, re-listening to the tapes with the transcript (typed by a professional) can also achieve this.

Working with the data

Crafting stories

In the midst of my doctoral journey I attended a workshop run by Max van Manen where he talked of crafting the data. I had a prejudice that data was sacrosanct, that to change one word was to undermine it in some way. We were sent away to craft a story from one of our own transcripts. I plunged into the challenge. The transcript I had with me had been of poor recording quality. It had words missing. It was messy. However, as I flicked through the pages I saw a story emerge. Plucking words from here and there, over four pages of transcript, not to change them, but to draw them together to recreate an evocative 'telling' yielded this story:

> We left coming home too late in the day. My husband was late get-ting there and I wasn't organised. Dressing a newborn baby into all her beautiful baby clothes was just a nightmare, like there were rib-bons on everything. I couldn't bend her arms into the gown. The baby was pretty upset by the time it was all done. I remember being really concerned about how cold it was. We had a debate about where to put the bassinette. I managed to last until we got to the front door and then I burst into tears and the feeling of 'what have we done, what on earth have we done and how on earth are we going to be able to do this?' When we got into the house it was just overwhelming. I remem-ber quite a few tears over that, just sort of thinking gosh, I have no idea about being a mother and here I am with full responsibility for a little mite. It was just so scary.

(Author)

From that point on, I crafted all my transcripts into stories. It is the stories that are returned to participants to ensure that in the re-crafting the mean-ing has remained 'as it was'. I now see that the crafting of data honours the participants for the meaning they have shared. Words are packaged in a manner that is easy to read, without embarrassing grammatical lapses. The writing can become a precious account for them to keep. For the researcher, there are now distinct stories that stay in one's mind rather than pages and pages of transcripts. My research students often give each story a name, thereby having a handle by which to reach back and grab a story. Nevertheless, one needs to be mindful that the initial title may not be what the story is really about. A useful reference is Caelli (2001).

The order of things

In writing this chapter I make it look as though one first does the interviews and then moves on to data analysis. That is not the case. The following paragraphs need to be read hand-in-hand with this one. Ideally, one does an interview, transcribes it, crafts the stories, writes the initial analysis and then moves on to the next interview with those thoughts fresh in one's ask-ing/listening/thinking. In reality one is likely to have two or perhaps three participants all somewhere in the process at the same time. What is to be avoided is collecting all the data and then beginning the analysis. Not only do you lose the opportunity to take thinking to the on-going interviews, but you are likely to feel overwhelmed by the sudden mass of words. Dwelling with a transcript before engaging closely with the next gives each its very own thinking space.

Analysing in a hermeneutic/interpretive manner

It is at this stage of the process that the hermeneutic phenomenological lens needs to explicitly show itself. There is a tendency for researchers to assume that as long as the data are telling stories of experience, identifying themes makes it phenomenology. A simple thematic analysis is not enough, yet in itself it is an appropriate methodological approach. It just needs to be named as 'Descriptive interpretive research' rather than carry the label of phenomenology. To choose to do hermeneutic interpretive phenomenology one needs to understand and demonstrate skills of interpretation. This is a useful time to turn to philosophers who interpret the writings of Heidegger and Gadamer, such as Dreyfus (2001), Grondin (1991), Harman (2007), Large (2008), Inwood (1997), Schmidt (2006), Wrathall (2005), and Young (1997). Turn also to writings of researchers who offer their own interpretation of how such philosophy is translated into method (Dowling 2004, Mackey 2005, Smythe *et al.* 2008, van Manen 1990). All of these will point you back to the classic philosophical texts of Heidegger and Gadamer. If you are a doctoral student you will need to move on to the original source, texts such as Heidegger's *Being and Time* (1995), Gadamer's *Truth and Method* (1982) and whatever else usefully informs your data analysis.

The nature of the thinking

One needs to grasp the nature of thinking called for in this kind of research. Harman (2007, p. 155) reminds us that: 'Phenomenology means a way of staying true to what must be thought'. Thinking is the interpretative act which brings understanding, which is thinking, which is interpretation – there is no linear progression to an end point, rather a lived experience of dwelling with the possibilities of what something could mean. Hermeneutic phenomenological thinking is not something done in one's 'mind' in a logical, systematic manner. Heidegger suggests thinking already has a mood; we are already perplexed, or anxious, or dismissive. We are already drawn to a particular part of the story; already sensing what matters; already overlooking the taken-for-granted.

Understanding 'Dasein'

Understanding 'Dasein' is fundamental to grasping the nature of such thinking. Heidegger's use of this German word is not readily translated to

English, which results in it being 'held' in its original language. Its etymological meaning is 'being there' (Heidegger 1995, p. 27). Sheehan (2001) suggests another interpretation: 'openness'. Let me try to explain. Right now you are reading this book. You are reading it 'somewhere', on a favourite chair, in a train, in your office, sitting in a café. There may be people around you, distracting you, or offering the opportunity to share thoughts as you read. Other people may be called to mind, drawing you to think 'I wish she was here so I could...'. In absence, people also bring their presence. Your body will be engaged in this process of reading, maybe in a forgetful manner, not intruding at all. Or maybe you forgot your glasses and your eyes feel like they are straining. Growing hunger might announce that it is time to think about finding food. Time ticks on through this experience. Your half hour of spare time might have disappeared in a flash. Or you might be sitting in an airport waiting, waiting, waiting for a delayed plane, each hour seeming endless. The point is, you are never just 'reading'. You are always reading in a context that influences the experience in a myriad of ways. Dasein, being-there, always 'is'. In so 'being' you are always open to the things/thoughts/feelings/people that 'call' and forgetful or ignorant of all else that is 'there' but does not claim your attention. Other methodologies may seek to remove the issue from its complex context. Phenomenology, in contrast, accepts that not only can we never escape context but that the 'there' of being makes the experience what it 'is'.

The hermeneutic 'as'

Another way of considering such an approach is through what is called the hermeneutic 'as'. Nothing is ever simply a 'thing'. You are reading this book 'as' a means to 'pass a tedious assignment', 'prepare a proposal', 'do a teaching session' – each of which will draw you to read in a different way, with a different sense of eagerness. Later, this book may find its 'as' as a gift to a friend who needs it more than you, a symbol on your bookshelf reminding you of this time in your life, or perhaps a doorstop. It is never just a book. The day it becomes the means by which to light a fire, its bookness becomes something quite different. Data analysis is about discerning the 'as', which may open possibilities that reveal new meaning. A book is never just as book. It is always a book 'as'...

Resonance

As you read, be it the data or the philosophical texts, some bits may cause you to mark them so you can return to them later, while other bits you will just skim. Some bits of data will quickly become 'favourite' and others discarded as being irrelevant, or not striking enough, or repetitive of what other people have said better. In openness, we are always open to some things while other things pass us by, almost, or entirely, unnoticed.

We notice what matters to us. That is why I am writing about these philosophical notions in this part of the chapter rather than at the beginning. When one starts to do one's own research, reading philosophy is of interest but in an ontic sort of a way; as theory, as ideas that have no feel of personal connection. It is when one begins to dwell with the data, to ponder meaning, to ask questions, that the philosophy comes alive. As someone who has been grappling with these philosophical texts over many years, in each new study as I read familiar works, lines jump off the page that previously I passed over. With fresh questions in my thinking, I find myself marking sections of the book previously left pristine. Such resonance is at the heart of hermeneutic interpretive thinking.

Trusting the process

In such a reading, thinking, pondering journey one needs to develop the confidence to read what one does not yet understand, and keep reading on through the fog. It may be that one phrase will suddenly open a doorway to insight; or as you put the book down (or data, because the reading of one will inform the reading of the other) and wander off you may find that your thoughts have moved on in an imperceptible way that leads you forward. Trust the process.

Living the method

I am not suggesting that you find a philosophical notion and then look for some data that matches. The data itself must always drive the research. First you dwell with each story, and in the dwelling flick through the philosophical texts in the hope that resonance will come when you read something that helps you make an interpretive leap. The leap enables you to say something more than what the participants said themselves; to uncover the meaning from between the lines, from behind the saying. This is the doing-everything-together phase of the study. You are dwelling closely with your data, and reading, and writing, and talking with your supervisor, and going back to your data, re-writing, still reading, still thinking, still letting the thoughts come.

Writing and re-writing

When I first met the term re-writing perhaps I assumed it was a kind of edit. I certainly had no conception of the nature of the research journey ahead of me. I had not yet grasped that the way to 'think' was to write. I began the process of writing through the data, taking each story and writing what I thought it might mean. I had identified themes which broke the writing into chapter sized chunks. One day I realized I had 13 such chapters. In the back of my mind I knew that a research report usually has three or four data chapters.

There was clearly a problem. Looking back I see that this was not a problem at all; this is what it means to write and re-write. Fortunately, at that juncture, I attended a phenomenological workshop run by Professors Nancy and John Diekelmann. Their question to me was: 'what are the three things that matter most?'. After a much needed holiday I sat down at my desk. In a flash I saw that I already knew what those three chapters would be: 1) that safety or unsafety is always already there; 2) however, there is a spirit of safe practice that can make practice safer; and 3) that relationships matter but are not the most important thing. I had the 'thesis of my thesis' because I had done the writing/thinking/reading to show myself my understandings. This was different to a simple thematic analysis. This was uncovering understanding towards building an argument. My challenge then, and in subsequent publications, was to take the reader with me so s/he too could come to understand the thinking that had emerged from the data.

An example of data analysis

First dwell with the data

First dwell with the data. The research question I brought to my doctorate was 'what is the meaning of being safe?' That is the question that one needs to keep firmly to the front of one's thinking. Pay attention to what grabs you as you read this story:

> It was a homebirth. The woman had made no progress at all. Her sister was fluffing around. I didn't pick it up right away that that's what the problem was, because her sister was being very attentive. And so eventually her labour stopped. I took the woman aside and I said 'well, what's the problem', and she said 'well, it's my sister and I can't ask her to go home'. I said 'I'll ask her to go home', so I explained to her that labour had stopped and it would probably be a good idea if she went home and let the woman have a rest. What it turned out was, that this girl had been sexually abused by her brother, and when she had told her sister, the sister denied this could have happened to her. So there was all this hostility between them. As soon as her sister went, away went labour and she had a nice normal birth. So you see, just changing that factor made the difference. Otherwise what are you going to do, are you going to transfer?
>
> (A – midwife)

When I read this I was struck by the breadth of thinking of this midwife. In a hospital setting 'failure to progress' is likely to have brought thoughts of augmentation. Instead, this homebirth midwife sensed there was a problem, but she did not know what. In a matter-of-fact way she talks of asking the woman what the problem was. I wondered how often that happens. What is startlingly revealed in this story is that the woman knew exactly what the problem was. Note what happened then – the woman said she couldn't ask her sister to leave. The midwife did not say 'shall I ask her for you?' Rather, she took control of the situation, thereby removing the 'problem'.

Resonance from reading

At the time of talking to this midwife, my reading of Heidegger had connected with the notions of care and solicitude. This had resonance with the story set out above. With this in mind, I began the chapter in which this piece of data was eventually set with the following reflection (abbreviated):

> From the word 'solicitude' Heidegger goes on to describe two extreme possibilities of its positive mode. He describes 'leaping in' as taking away 'care' from the other, taking over for the other. King (1964, p. 107) interprets this as when someone (for example, the practitioner) 'leaps in' they take 'care' off the other, usually by taking care of things for them (for example, taking care of a woman's decisions by telling her what will happen). …On the other hand, there may be times when in the need to be safe, the practitioner must leap in with their own decision of what needs to happen. In 'leaping-in' care of the woman becomes dominated by 'what the practitioner thinks is best'… 'Leaping ahead', in contrast, goes ahead of the other, not to take away their care but to give it back to them. It helps the other [the woman] see themselves in their care, and become 'free for it".
>
> (Heidegger 1962/1927, p. 159)

Understanding is always within its own context. In New Zealand in the 1990s when I was writing this thesis, midwives had just become able to practise in their own right and were advocating a philosophical model of partnership where all decisions were made 'with' the woman. Here was Heidegger saying that sometimes in 'care' decisions are 'taken away' from the other person. It is such resonance of understanding that reveals disconnects, bringing forth the thinking of this methodological approach.

Making an interpretive leap

As I dwelt with this story I saw afresh the interplay of leaping-ahead and leaping-in. When the midwife asked the woman what the problem was she was 'leaping ahead' (as fitting to a philosophy of partnership) in an extraordinary way, believing that this woman would understand why her contractions had gone off. However, when the woman said she could not ask her sister to leave, this midwife 'leapt in'. She took that decision away from the woman. She gave the woman no choice. The authority of that moment was the midwife's. Yet, the spirit of the leaping-in was to free the woman to again leap-ahead in being able to continue to labour safely at home.

Coming to 'see'

I came to see that safe practice was about more than 'partnership'. It was a relationship of trust that meant the midwife was free to 'leap in' to keep the situation safe. Yes, 'leaping ahead' is preferable, but in itself it may not be sufficient. I came to understand the complex nature of the play of safe practice. It is unlikely I would have achieved the depth of this analysis without the insights I gleaned from reading Heidegger.

The thinking goes on

As I go back to this story ten years later I am struck by what still lies hidden. In a thesis that asked about the meaning of being safe in childbirth, here is a pointer that a history of sexual abuse and all the subsequent lack of trust that emerges from such an experience have been left silent in my analysis. I recognize that I was more focused on 'practising safely', yet from a woman's perspective I now see that I needed to recognize more clearly that safety in childbirth can be undermined years before the woman becomes pregnant. That is the unfolding, revealing nature of the experience of analysis. One starts by seeing what immediately captures one's attention. And yes, one does need to stay very focused on the particular interest. Each story has so many different avenues of exploration. There is never an end. Perhaps now as I work with a student exploring the experience of women who have a history of sexual abuse my own horizon has changed. I am now more open to 'thinking'. I share this to alert you to the need to do analysis slowly, to return to it time and time again, to submit the research report knowing there is still much of the meaning hidden and untold.

Pulling it all together

Your writing and re-writing will lead you to a concise argument that will articulate the meaning of your chosen phenomenon. In writing your report the data always need to lead: take the reader to the experience, point to what you see, and then invite them to think along with you. Other methodologies tend to 'tell' – they explain their ideas to the reader and then back them up with an example from the data. In hermeneutic interpretive phenomenology the data (the nearest we can document of the primordial experience) always drive. It is followed by the researcher's own interpretations and then some philosophical notions or relevant references may be offered to join in play with the thinking. The hallmark of having got to some sort of 'end' is when someone asks you to describe the meaning of your phenomenon and you can do that in a five-minute statement. However, the watermark of phenomenology is when a story read from the data holds the audience in an almost sacred silence. They are captured by a felt knowing that stays with them in a story that becomes their own.

The remainder of the research project

Chapter one

Once the data chapters are completed it is time to go back to the beginning of the research report. The introduction (which is often begun early in the journey but finished off towards the end) offers a clearly stated research question, describes the impetus for the study, gives background context, argues for the choice of methodology and outlines the structure of the research report.

The literature review

The literature review is usually also conducted in this later time slot. You will have been gathering and reading related literature, and will have identified an initial 'gap' to support your study, but now is the time for some different thinking. At this end of your research report you will have become skilled in hermeneutic analysis. The lens you brought to your data is the same lens you need to bring to the literature. In my study on the meaning of 'being safe' just about every article ever written about childbirth could have been relevant to the study. My experience as a supervisor suggests there is often an overwhelming feast of related literature, yet a famine of anything that closely relates to the experience itself. Once you have come to see your argument, you will be drawn to explore literature that earlier you may not have considered relevant. All your reading will now be through the lens of the thinking that has emerged through your research journey. The purpose of your literature review is not simply to show the existing literature but rather to portray the taken-for-granted meanings that make up the knowing of practice. Further, it is to engage in another layer of thinking. As a hermeneutic scholar you will always read with your own understandings revealing agreement and difference. Where there is another view, perhaps because of context, historical time, culture, or paradigm, such difference opens up new possibilities for thinking. Reading outside of midwifery literature will similarly open up wider horizons of thinking. Poetry, novels, or any of the more artistic genres may bring you gems. For example, lines from a poem by Walt Whitman enabled me to discern the meaning of what I called the spirit of safe practice:

> Have you heard that it was good to gain the day?
> I also say it is good to fall,
> battles are lost in the same spirit in which they are won.
> (*Song of Myself,* Walt Whitman, 1855)

Methodology/method

Next you need to write the methodology/method section. Again you may have started this earlier but usually it does not have sufficient depth of understanding until the research journey has been lived. The method section/chapter needs to tell your own story of how you conducted the research and offer the reader criteria against which you argue your study is trustworthy (Davies and Dodd 2002, de Witt and Ploeg 2006, Emden and Sandelowski 1999, Koch 1996, 1999, 2006).

Conclusion

In the final paragraph you need to do more than simply summarize your findings. This is where the 'parts' become a whole, which is always more than a summation of parts. You articulate the thesis of your research report (your argument); you tell the story of how the phenomenon of the study is lived. And in keeping with the methodology you point to all that is still not yet known.

Final reflections

There is no end to hermeneutic interpretive phenomenology, just a time of offering a report in some form, knowing that there is much still unthought and unsaid. The examiner or reviewer of such research will be looking for philosophical congruence that pervades the entire work. They will be attuned to the resonance of your interpretive analysis. The hallmark of excellence is to draw them into their own thinking. Revealing the rich, complex, dynamic, mysterious, nature of being human brings a gift to self. As one comes to understand others, one learns to see, to think and to be attuned in a more attentive way. Perhaps one becomes wise; yet paradoxically one is left feeling humble.

To choose hermeneutic interpretive phenomenology to guide one's research is to open oneself to a journey of thinking, where thoughts 'come' and knowing emerges. It is to re-connect with what it means to be human, and discover afresh what is already known, but perhaps forgotten, hidden or put aside. It is to expose vulnerability and resilience, dread and hope, sadness and joy. It is to celebrate and despair. But always it is to remember what matters; to strive to enhance the experience of those we go on to walk with through similar experiences. Yes, a phenomenon has been articulated, but always it comes back to people, people like you and me. Life is only ever lived as 'my experience'.

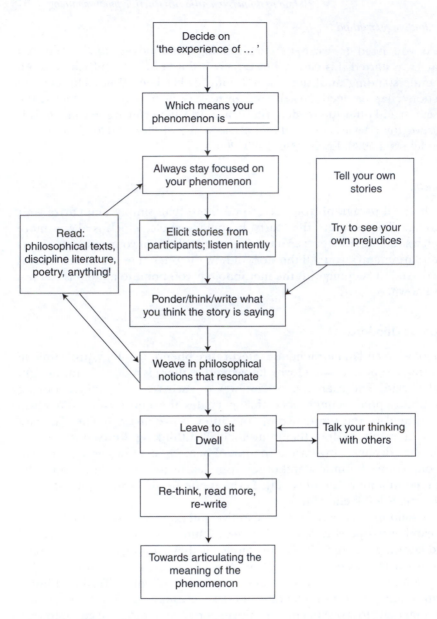

Figure 3.1 A glimpse of the hermeneutic interpretive phenomenological process: always in motion, never linear, always going back-and-forth-and-around

References

Caelli K. (2001) Engaging with Phenomenology: Is it More of a Challenge than it Needs to be? *Qualitative Health Research* 11, 273–281.

Collins J. (2000) *Heidegger and the Nazis.* Icon: Cambridge.

Davies D. and Dodd J. (2002) Qualitative Research and the Question of Rigor *Qualitative Health Research* 12, 279–289.

de Witt L. and Ploeg J. (2006) Critical appraisal of rigour in interpretive phenomenological nursing research. *Journal of Advanced Nursing* 55, 215–229.

Dowling M. (2004) Hermeneutics: an exploration. *International Journal of Nursing Studies* 11, 30–40.

Dreyfus H. (2001) *Being-in-the-World.* The MIT Press: London.

Emden C. and Sandelowski M. (1999) The good, the bad and the relative, part two: Goodness and the criterion problem in qualitative research. *International Journal of Nursing Studies* 5, 2–7.

Fiumara G. C. (1990) *Midwifery and Philosophy. The Other Side of Language: A Philosophy of Listening.* Routledge: New York.

Gadamer H. G. (1982) *Truth and Method* (G. Barden and J. Cumming, trans.). Crossroad: New York.

Gadamer H. G. (2007) *The Gadamer Reader* (R. E. Palmer, trans.). Northwestern University Pres: Evanston, Illinois.

Grondin J. (1991) *Introduction to Philosophical Hermeneutics.* Yale University Press: New Haven.

Harman G. (2007) *Heidegger Explained.* Open Court: Chicago.

Heidegger M. (1962/1927) *Being and Time* (J. McQuarrie and E. Robinson, trans.). Basil Blackwell: Oxford.

Heidegger M. (1995) *Being and Time* (J. McQuarrie and E. Robinson, trans.). Basil Blackwell: Open Court.

Inwood M. (1997) *Heidegger.* Oxford Paperbacks: Oxford.

King M. (1964) *Heidegger's Philosophy: A Guide to his Basic Thought.* Basil Blackwell: Oxford.

Koch T. (1996) Implementation of a hermeneutic inquiry in nursing: philosophy, rigour and representation. *Journal of Advanced Nursing* 24, 174–184.

Koch T. (1999) An interpretive research process: revisiting phenomenological and hermeneutic approaches. *Nurse Researcher* 6, 20–34.

Koch T. (2006) Establishing rigour in qualitative research: the decision trail. *Journal of Advanced Nursing* 53, 91–103.

Lang B. (1996) *Heidegger's Silence.* Cornell University Press: Ithaca.

Large W. (2008) *Heidegger's Being and Time.* Indiana University Press: Bloomington.

Mackey S. (2005) Phenomenological nursing research: methodological insights derived from Heidegger's interpretive phenomenology. *International Journal of Nursing Studies* 42, 179–186.

Schmidt L. (2006) *Understanding Hermeneutics.* Acumen: Stocksfield.

Sheehan T. (2001) A Paradigm shift in Heidegger research. *Continental Philosophy Review*, XXXII, 1–20.

Smythe E. (1998) *'Being Safe' in Childbirth: A Hermeneutic Interpretation of the Narratives of Women and Practitioners.* Unpublished PhD, Massey University: Auckland.

Smythe E. (2003) Uncovering the meaning of 'being safe' in practice. *Contemporary Nurse* 14, 196–204.

Smythe E., Ironside P., Sims S., Swenson M. and Spence, D. (2008) Doing Heideggerian hermeneutic research: A discussion paper. *International Journal of Nursing Studies* 45, 1389–1397.

van Manen M. (1990) *Researching Lived Experience.* The Althouse Press: London, Ontario.

Whitman W. (1855) *Song of Myself, 18.* In *The Works of Walt Whitman.* Wordsworth Editions: Hertfordshire.

Wrathall M. (2005) *Heidegger.* Granta Books: London.

Young J. (1997) *Heidegger, Philosophy, Nazism.* Cambridge University Press: Cambridge.

4 Phenomenological research approaches
Mapping the terrain of competing perspectives

Maura Dowling

Introduction

There are many phenomenological approaches, and understanding the differences and subtleties between these approaches is important. However, it is no simple task. 'It is doubtful whether any article, or even a single book, could describe sufficiently all the nuances and complete evolution of phenomenology' (Gearing 2004, p. 1430). Moreover, the historical setting from which phenomenology emerged is 'extraordinarily complex and hence open to a variety of interpretations' (Zaner and Ihde 1973, p. 12).

Spiegelberg (1971/1965) argues, 'for better or worse, the underlying assumption of a unified philosophy subscribed to by all as so-called phenomenologists is an illusion. Besides, "phenomenologists" are much too individualistic in their habits to form an organized "school"' (p. xxxvii). He also adds that the varieties of phenomenology 'exceed the common features' (Spiegelberg 1971/1965, p. xxxvii).

The many phenomenological research approaches proposed illustrate the popularity of this research movement. This is not surprising in view of the huge potential of phenomenology. In an attempt to explain this potential, the following is useful: 'Just as fish may take for granted the water they swim in, we as humans may find it difficult to notice and articulate the humanly qualitative nature of the world we live in' (Todres *et al.* 2007, p. 54). Phenomenology helps us notice and articulate this world.

Essentially, phenomenology looks for answers to the question, 'How do we know?' (Ray 1994, p. 118), and aims to 'turn toward phenomena which have been blocked from sight by the theoretical patterns in front of them'. In terms of phenomenology as a research approach, Dahlberg *et al.* (2001) offer a clear description of phenomenology's role. In order for researchers to 'go to the things themselves', researchers 'stand in such a way that the things can show themselves to us, and thus "the thing" is understood as a phenomenon' (Dahlberg *et al.* 2001, p. 45).

This chapter traces the origins of the philosophy of phenomenology and maps the movement of phenomenology from a philosophy to a research approach, through the initial work undertaken by those aligned to the

Duquesne school. Husserl's central role in the phenomenological movement is threaded throughout the chapter and the various approaches to phenomenological research, including descriptive, lifeworld and interpretive/ hermeneutic phenomenology are charted. The popularity of phenomenological styles that adopt a mixture of approaches is also discussed.

Origins of phenomenology

Phenomenology emerged in the late nineteenth century in a challenge to the then dominant positivist view of philosophy and psychology (Ehrich 2005). The term 'phenomenology' is derived from the Greek words of 'phainoemn' (appearance) and 'logos' (reason) (Gearing 2004). The first documented use of the term 'phenomenology' was by Johann Heinrich Lambert in 1764 (Spiegelberg 1971/1965). It was then used by philosophy texts in the eighteenth century, especially by Kant and later by Hegel, who made the most prominent use of the term when it featured in the title of his 1807 work *Phenomenology of Spirit* (Moran 2000). However, the inspiration for Husserl's use of the term 'phenomenology' was neither Kant nor Hegel, but Franz Brentano (Moran 2000). Brentano (1838–1917), a psychologist and philosopher, used the phrase 'descriptive psychology or descriptive phenomenology' and revived the medieval notion of 'intentionality'. It was while attending Brentano's lectures in Vienna that Husserl's intellectual path to phenomenology was paved (Cerbone 2006). It was also Brentano who influenced Husserl to shift from mathematics to philosophy (Crotty 1996).

The terms 'intentionality', 'noema' and 'noesis' are central concepts in phenomenology which 'are fraught with complexity' (Moustakas 1994, p. 68). Husserl adopted Brentano's account of 'intentionality' as the fundamental concept for understanding and classifying conscious acts and experiential mental practices (Moustakas 1994). Husserl referred to the 'presentational function of consciousness', where 'consciousness actualizes presences' (Giorgi 2005, p. 76). Intentionality relates to the 'union of object and subject' (Crotty 1996, p. 42), and is based on the principle that every mental act is related to some object (Moran 2000), and implies that all perceptions have meaning (Owen 1994). All thinking, including 'imagining, perceiving, remembering etc.' is always thinking about something (van Manen 1990, p. 182). Intentionality therefore refers to 'a principle of openness' (Giorgi 2005, p. 76), and to the internal experience of being conscious of something, 'whether actually existing or not' (Moustakas 1994, p. 68).

Noema refers to that which is experienced, and noesis refers to the way it is experienced: 'when we look at something what we see intuitively constitutes its meaning' (Moustakas 1994, p. 70). Crotty (1996) further explains this by outlining that 'phenomenological analysis involves both the act of the subject (the *noetic* dimension) and the content or object of the act (the *noematic* dimension)' (p. 33).

Husserl's phenomenological project

Prior to the Second World War, phenomenology was mainly a German event and all discussions on phenomenology have their origins in the philosophy of phenomenology espoused by Edmund Husserl (1859–1938) (Spiegelberg 1971/1965). As mentioned above, excited by the work of Franz Brentano in 'descriptive psychology', in the period 1900–1901, Husserl proclaimed that phenomenology was '…a bold, radically new way of doing philosophy, an attempt to bring philosophy back from abstract metaphysical speculation wrapped in pseudo-problems, in order to come into contact with the matters themselves, with concrete living experience' (Moran 2000, p. xiii). (Also refer to Bondas, Chapter 1 for further insights into Husserlian descriptive phenomenology.)

Husserl plays a central role in the phenomenological movement. Ricoeur (1967) argues that: 'All of phenomenology is not Husserl, even though he is more or less its center' (p. 3). Other philosophers associated with phenomenology include Hans-Georg Gadamer, Maurice Merleau-Ponty, Hannah Arendt, Emmanuel Levinas, John-Paul Sarte, and Jacques Derrida (Moran 2000). Moreover, the work of Alfred Schutz on phenomenological psychology also had its influence from Husserl's transcendental phenomenology (Embree 2008). The influence of Hannah Arendt is also noteworthy to this text. Although Arendt has been acknowledged for her writings on identity, she was not acknowledged for her work on gender.

An early follower of Husserl was Johannes Daubert (a student of Theodor Lipps in Munich), who met with Husserl in 1902. Husserl subsequently visited Munich and met with a group of Lipps' students. The outcome of this gathering was the establishment of the Munich Phenomenological Circle which signalled 'the birth of the phenomenological movement' (Crotty 1996, p. 53).

Phenomenological attitude

Husserl 'sought a philosophy without presuppositions' (Cohen and Omery 1994, p. 138). He argued that phenomenology leads us 'back to the things themselves' (zu den Sachen selbst) before we apply our pre-understandings; therefore phenomenology 'aims to demonstrate how the world is an *experience which we live* before it becomes an *object which we know* in some impersonal or detached fashion' (Kearney 1994, p. 13).

Husserl's mantra that we should 'go back to the things themselves' involved moving outside our everyday experience ('natural attitude'), by adopting a 'phenomenological attitude'. The 'phenomenological attitude' is considered to be probably the most important aspect of phenomenological research (Finlay 2008). The process involves an attempt to suspend presuppositions and look at the world anew while employing a reflexive stance to hold pre-understandings in abeyance. 'It is not our experience after we have developed or applied ways of understanding and explaining it. It is experience as it is before we have thought about it' (Crotty 1996, p. 53).

Husserl uses the term 'natural' to indicate what is original, naïve, prior to critical or theoretical reflection (van Manen 1990):

> [In the] natural attitude, one is immersed in, and thus in a sense lost in the usual activity...we do not consider it necessary to analyze those things which are closest and which seem obvious, that is, our tacit or implicit experiencing of the world.
>
> (Dahlberg *et al.* 2001, p. 46)

In the natural attitude individuals hold knowledge judgementally but epoché requires a fresh way of looking at things (Moustakas 1994). 'Epoché' is a Greek word meaning to refrain from judgement or avoid the everyday, commonplace way of perceiving things (Moustakas 1994). However, in order to bracket one's preconceptions and presuppositions, one must firstly know them (Valle *et al.* 1989). Husserl describes this as: 'A new way of experiencing, thinking, of theorizing...', where '...all natural interests are put out of play...' (Husserl 1970/1936, p. 152).

Phenomenological reduction follows epoché (Moustakas 1994). It allows us to be 'led back to the origins of phenomena: these origins are lost in the haste of our everyday thought' (Cohen and Omery 1994, p. 136). Gearing (2004) argues that, although there are underlying philosophical differences between the terms 'phenomenological reduction', 'epoché' and 'bracketing', they are often referred to simultaneously to reflect the 'similarity of their core essences' (p. 1430). However, Husserl's writings on phenomenological reduction or bracketing evolved during his writings and 'has remained openly definable in certain of its core elements' (Gearing 2004, p. 1430).

Phenomenological reduction

Husserl proposed a number of 'reductions', one of which was transcendental reduction (Finlay 2008). Husserl believed that reduction freed us from our previous understandings thus allowing us to see things as they were. Spiegelberg (1982/1965) argues that 'phenomenological intuiting' is at the heart of phenomenological reduction. This involves the phenomenologist attempting to meet the phenomenon in as free and unprejudiced a way as possible, in order that the phenomenon may present itself in as free and unprejudiced a way as possible so that it can be precisely described and understood.

However, this aspect of phenomenology generates much confusion and many papers debate how it can be achieved (e.g. Lowes and Prowse 2001, LeVasseur 2003). It 'frequently appears as methodologically superficial or vague' (Gearing 2004, p. 1429). Moreover, some phenomenological studies are accused of 'inappropriately and erroneously reducing bracketing to a formless technique, value stance, or black-box term' (Gearing 2004, p. 1432).

The utilization of reduction, according to Giorgi (1985) means that the phenomenological researcher takes the meaning of any experience as it presents itself or appears in consciousness. 'What appears in consciousness is the phenomenon' (Moustakas 1994, p. 26). Many techniques are recommended in pursuit of reduction; the most popular being the identification and articulation of assumptions prior to data collection and analysis (Cohen and Omery 1994, Ray 1994). However, Finlay (2008) warns that novice researchers commonly misinterpret the bracketing process of merely identifying and setting aside presuppositions, thus under-appreciating the 'complexity and discipline of the phenomenological attitude as a whole' (p. 3). Finlay (2008) proposes a view of the phenomenological attitude that 'does not involve a researcher who is striving to be objectivistic, distanced or detached. Instead, the researcher is fully involved, interested and open to what might appear' (p. 3).

McNamara (2005) discusses useful insights on the issue of intentionality and study participants (co-researchers). Drawing on Crotty's (1996) five-step method for doing phenomenology, McNamara details how in his interviewing with study participants, he adopted the role of 'midwife to her [sic] co-researchers as they labour to cast received notions aside in order to look at the phenomenon anew' (McNamara 2005, p. 698).

Transition from a philosophy to a research approach

Wilson (2002) applauds the significance of phenomenology to the social sciences and highlights how Husserl's ideas, amended and developed, have informed research approaches in sociology, psychology, education, health sciences, and many other disciplines. How did the theoretical writings of Husserl and others develop over the twentieth century to become a major force in qualitative research? Kearney (1994) argues that French phenomenologists (Sarte, Merleau-Ponty and Ricoeur) succeeded in rendering phenomenology 'more accessible and engaging' (p. 12) and the translation of phenomenology from German into French extended 'its range of relevance' (p. 12).

Merleau Ponty (1908–1961) proposed that phenomenology is best appreciated in the context of the phenomenological method, which he argues has four key characteristics: it is descriptive, it utilizes reduction, it searches for essences and it is focused on the intentionality (De Castro 2003). These four key qualities, or 'celebrated themes' are common to different types of phenomenology (Ehrich 2005, p. 2).

In relation to phenomenology as a research endeavour, all types of phenomenological research generally utilize one or more sources for its data. These sources of data include: a) the researcher's reflection on his/her own experience(s) pertaining to the phenomenon under investigation; b) the study participants' verbal or written accounts of their experiences of the phenomenon under investigation; and c) descriptions of the phenomenon gleaned from literature, visual art, poetry, electronic media, performing arts, and other phenomenological research (Hein and Austin 2001). Hermeneutic phenomenology methods generally rely on the third data source just outlined (Hein and Austin 2001). The utilization of poetry as 'data' is illustrated in a study of midwives' way of knowing during childbirth reported by Hunter (2008). Poems written by ten midwives were used for the study's data. (Further interpretations of poetry are presented by Hunter in Chapter 10.)

Psychological investigators in the early twentieth century were drawn towards phenomenology. A successful branch of psychology subsequently developed known as phenomenological psychology (Wilson 2002). The movement of phenomenology into psychology was facilitated principally by the work of Giorgi (1985, 1994), Polkinghorne (1989), Moustakas (1994) and van Kaam (1959, 1966). However, it is important to highlight that phenomenological psychology is not a subfield of the phenomenological philosophy movement; it is a branch of psychology that draws direction from philosophy (Polkinghorne 1989, Hein and Austin 2001).

Descriptive/Husserlian phenomenology

van Kaam is considered the founder of descriptive or 'empirical phenomenology'; so-called because of its rigorous approach to data collection and analysis (Hein and Austin 2001). van Kaam's doctoral dissertation, completed in 1958, was a study which asked 365 high school seniors and college students to describe a situation (or situations) where they felt truly understood by another person (Hein and Austin 2001). This study appears to map the juncture where phenomenological philosophy crossed over to phenomenological research.

During the 1970s, two university departments (the psychology department of the University of Duquesne, Pittsburgh, and the department of education at the University of Götenborg, Sweden) were pursuing qualitative approaches as an alternative to the empirical method (Giorgi 1986). Amendo Giorgi was faculty member of the psychology department of Duquesne University, a department 'wholly committed to the phenomenological method in psychology', where the term 'Duquesne method' was used to describe their approach (Giorgi 2008, p. 34). Giorgi's approach, labelled 'scientific phenomenology', adapts Husserl's philosophical method, and also is inspired by some of Merleau-Ponty's (1962) insights in his pursuit of a method that 'could be used for studying psychological phenomena within a scientific context' (Giorgi 2008, p. 34). Giorgi's method is considered 'as close a translation as possible of Husserl's phenomenological method' (Smith *et al.* 2009, p. 200). Moreover, his phenomenological research method is also known as an 'existential phenomenological method' because of its adoption of Merleau-Ponty's views (De Castro 2003).

The label of the 'Duquesne school' is used loosely because the entire original group who worked at Duquesne university did not remain there

(Cohen and Omery 1994, p. 150). The Duquesne school considers the phenomenological method to include description, adoption of phenomenological reduction, and disclosure of essences as results (Garza 2007). Others attributed to the Duquesne school include Colaizzi, Fisher and van Kaam (Cohen and Omery 1994), and their work assumed a dominant position in the phenomenological movement (Hein and Austin 2001). More recently, phenomenological research at the University of Dallas has followed the Duquesne school (Garza 2007).

Moustakas, also from the field of psychology, presents two phenomenological methods, one adapted from van Kaam's phenomenological method and the other from the Stevick-Colaizzi-Keen method (Moustakas 1994). The seven-step phenomenological method proposed by Moustakas (1994) has been popular among nursing and midwifery researchers. For instance, Peterson *et al.* (2007) used Moustakas' transcendental method to provide a description of adolescent mothers' perceptions of inpatient postpartum nursing care.

A characteristic of descriptive phenomenology is its focus on the structure of the phenomenon under scrutiny in order to reveal what is common to the different ways the phenomenon presents itself (Hein and Austin 2001). With this approach, the researcher steps out of their natural attitude and 'brackets' part of their world from consciousness. This is described by Giorgi (1997) as 'scientific phenomenological reduction'.

Free imaginative variation is also a feature of empirical phenomenology and used to illuminate the essences of a phenomenon. This process is described by Spiegelberg (1982/1965) as a type of mental experimentation during which the researcher intentionally uses his/her imagination to alter different aspects of the experience. Polkinghorne (1989, p. 55) argues that the purpose of this is to 'imaginatively stretch the proposed transformation to the edges until it no longer describes the experience underlying the subject's naive description'.

A rigorous process of data analysis is a key feature of descriptive phenomenology. Particular attention is paid to the research design and the steps taken in data analysis, which emphasizes the importance they place on rigour (Hein and Austin 2001). This rigorous process to data analysis is also evident in recent developments in phenomenology with the increasing popularity of Interpretative Phenomenological Analysis (IPA) (Smith *et al.* 2009). IPA, developed in psychology in the mid-1990s, and was mostly used in the UK in its early days (Smith *et al.* 2009) but is now utilized by a variety of disciplines worldwide. The increasing popularity of IPA reflects Polkinghorne's prediction that 'the translation of the philosophical methods developed by phenomenology into functioning research practices for psychology is unfinished' (Polkinghorne 1989, p. 43).

Another approach to existential-phenomenological research that has evolved from the University of Tennessee is that proposed by Pollio *et al.* (1997). Pollio *et al's* approach has been used by many nurse and midwife researchers, including Meighan *et al.* (1999), who describe the experiences of fathers living with a spouse with postpartum depression. Pollio *et al.'s* (1997) approach addresses the steps to be taken over the entire phenomenological study. Rather than providing steps for data analysis as with other approaches, such as that proposed by Colaizzi, Pollio *et al.'s* (1997) approach recommends that the researcher undergoes a bracketing interview in the early stage of their study. Ray (1994) also recommends the adoption of bracketing in descriptive phenomenology during the interview process. Research questions are therefore not predetermined. Similarly, Rolls and Relf (2004) also discuss the potential of bracketing interviews.

Descriptive phenomenology remains a popular approach for researchers in health related disciplines. For instance, Johansson and Berg (2005) describe their utilization of Giorgi's method 'based on Husserl's phenomenology with the lifeworld theory' (p. 58) in their study of women's experiences of childlessness two years after completing *in vitro* fertilization treatment. Colaizzi's phenomenological method is particularly popular. For instance, Chang and Mu (2008) utilize Colaizzi's approach in their study of the essential structure of family stress among hospitalized women receiving infertility treatment with ovarian hyper-stimulation syndrome. As did Clemmens (2002), who describes the postnatal depression experienced by adolescent mothers. Cheryl Beck has also utilized this methodology to explore women's postnatal mood and anxiety disorders (refer to Chapter 11). It is interesting that Colaizzi's method remains popular with midwife and nurse researchers, when Colaizzi has not remained active in phenomenological scholarship or debate. Thomas (2005, p. 66) regards this 'prolonged allegiance' by nurses with Colaizzi's method as 'puzzling'. However, Colaizzi's method does provide clear direction in its method and this is helpful to those new to phenomenological research.

The lifeworld ('lebenswelt')

The lifeworld, or 'lebenswelt', first articulated by Husserl, emerged from his views on the natural attitude (Dahlberg *et al.* 2001; also refer to Chapter 2). Husserl's work on the lifeworld emerged in the last decade of his life and is viewed as a signal to his rejection of his 'transcendental idealism' (Crotty 1996, p. 63). Husserl's 'parallel existence' of some of Heidegger's broad themes is also attributed to the influence of his assistant, Fink, whose philosophical creativity attempted to reconcile Husserl and Heidegger (Moran 2007, p. 13). Diekelmann (2001) argues that reflective lifeworld research illuminates what is similar and different between Husserl's transcendental phenomenology and Heidegger's hermeneutic phenomenology.

Husserl's concept of the 'lifeworld' produced by reduction also prompted Alfred Schutz (1899–1959) to propose an eradication of Husserl's distinction between 'lifeworld' and 'natural attitude' and to consider 'intersubjectivity as a given of everyday life' (Costelloe 1996, p. 247). Schutz laid the foundation for a phenomenological sociology (Wagner 1970), which resulted in phenomenology's huge impact on American sociology (Crotty 1996). Schutz's main concern was with 'what he called a phenomenology of the natural attitude carried out on the level of phenomenological psychology' (Natanson 1973, p. 26).

Discussions on the concept of 'lifeworld' are central to many phenomenological approaches (Berndtsson *et al.* 2007). Berndtsson *et al.* (2007) view the lifeworld in its ontological sense as 'the prereflective ground for our being in the world, which is given to us in the natural attitude and is taken for granted in everyday life' (p. 259). Moreover, with lifeworld research, 'the criteria of objectivity includes being as open as possible towards the phenomenon' (Johansson and Berg 2005, p. 59). Dahlberg *et al.* (2001) settle on a 'middle position' (p. 60) with regard to Husserl's notion of 'transcendentality', and argue on the impossibility of bracketing 'all pre-understandings in the world' (p. 61). With lifeworld research, Dahlberg and Dahlberg (2004) prefer to use the term 'bridling' instead of bracketing. They argue that bracketing carries with it an 'exactness and finitude of mathematics' (Dahlberg and Dahlberg 2004, p. 272) whereas 'bridling' also 'invokes the thought of being respectful, or humble, to that which is bridled in order not to dominate, violate it, or "swallow" it as "bracketing" seems to do' (p. 272).

Ashworth (1996) also proposed practical advice to researchers on how to bracket presuppositions in order for the lifeworld to reveal itself. He advised that researchers set aside their personal views and experience, scientific knowledge/explanations and truth or falsehood claims expressed by study participants.

Focus on the lifeworld seeks to illuminate its essential structures, and in doing so, has similarities with Giorgi's approach (Finlay 2009). However, while Ashworth's lifeworld phenomenological approach and IPA both seek out idiographic meanings, Giorgi's approach disregards idiographic details in favour of explicating the phenomenon as a whole (Finlay 2009). This is an interesting distinction because Crotty (1996) reminds us that it is not the aim of phenomenological research to illuminate shared meanings and disregard individual meanings unless they are also held by others.

Similar views on the lifeworld are expressed by Merleau-Ponty, Heidegger, Husserl and Gadamer (Dahlberg *et al.* 2001), who proposed 'intertwined' philosophical perspectives on the lifeworld, namely, temporality, spatiality, mood, embodiment and intersubjectivity (Biley and Galvin 2007, p. 802). Todres *et al.* (2007) also give an account of the lifeworld illustrating these five philosophical perspectives. Ashworth (2003) proposes seven interconnecting 'fractions' (p. 147) of the lifeworld, which are considered when undertaking data analysis and 'enables the detailed description of a given lifeworld to be undertaken in a thorough and phenomenological manner' (p. 147). The seven fragments (selfhood, sociality, embodiment, temporality, spatiality, project, discourse), outlined by Ashworth (2003) are drawn from Merleau-Ponty's *Phenomenology of Perception*. These seven fractions also bear a resemblance to van Manen's four lifeworld themes (existentials) of lived space (spatiality), lived body (corporeality), lived time (temporality) and lived human relation (relationality or communality) (van Manen 1990). Van Manen's approach is discussed in more depth later on in this chapter. Ashworth (2003) clarifies that each fragment 'will vary within a certain lifeworld' (p. 151). However, he also cautions that the fragments 'do not constitute a full account of the essence of lifeworld' (Ashworth 2003, p. 147).

Todres *et al.* (2007) also discuss Husserl's notion of the embodied lifeworld and using the dimensions of temporality, spatiality, intersubjectivity, embodiment and mood, argue its methodological potential 'How we live in relation to time, space, body, others and mood is fundamental to describing the holistic context in which being human makes sense' (Todres *et al.* 2007, p. 60).

For all lifeworld research, the researcher must 'engage in openness to the phenomenon' (Dahlberg *et al.* 2001, p. 96), and 'to be open means to conduct one's research on behalf of the phenomenon' (Dahlberg *et al.* 2001, p. 97). Finlay (2006) also proposes that researchers embrace openness in her phenomenological approach. She also argues that the challenge for researchers is to evaluate critically their pre-understandings during both the data collection and analysis phases and to create methods to manage their 'seductive power' (Finlay 2008, p. 17).

Dahlberg *et al.*'s (2001; see Chapter 2) approach to phenomenology draws its influence from both phenomenology and hermeneutics. Many studies have utilized this approach, including a study of midwives' experience of the encounter of women and their pain during childbirth (Lundgren and Dahlberg 2002); women's long-term memories of childbirth (refer to Chapter 7) and parents' participation in the care of their infant in the neonatal environment (refer to Chapter 9). IPA also draws on phenomenology and hermeneutics, but in conjunction with idiography (Smith *et al.* 2009).

IPA is also similar to van Manen's research method because it follows Husserl's call to return to experience itself and not attempt 'to fix experience in predefined or overly abstract categories' (Smith *et al.* 2009, p. 1), and is also an 'interpretative endeavour and is therefore informed by hermeneutics' (Smith *et al.* 2009, p. 3). Moreover, like IPA, van Manen's (1990) approach also searches for commonalities and differences in the textual descriptions of phenomena. IPA can also apply to one single case; an approach similar to that described by Greenwood and Lowenthal (2005) who utilize Bleicher's (1980) hermeneutic approach.

Interpretive/hermeneutic phenomenology

Husserl's work on the 'lifeworld' inspired other phenomenologists from the hermeneutic and existentialist traditions (Ehrich 2005). Husserl was always developing his views on fresh pathways, and with each new chapter in his thinking, his students developed his work further (Moran 2000). Moran (2000) therefore concludes that phenomenology is '...a historical movement...exemplified by a range of extraordinarily diverse thinkers' (Moran 2000, p. xiv).

Among these 'diverse thinkers' was Martin Heidegger (1889–1976), who transformed phenomenology through his rejection of Husserl's Cartesianism and transcendental idealism (Moran 2000). Heidegger accepted Husserl's views on phenomenology as returning 'to the things themselves' but where Husserl emphasized 'a consciousness-of-the-world', Heidegger viewed it as a 'being-in-the-world' (Kearney 1994, p. 30). Heidegger's ascent prompted the 'wounded' Husserl to 'reformulate his phenomenology' following the 'renewed vigour' he received from his loyal follower Fink (Moran 2007, p. 5). (For additional insights into Heidegger's philosophy and development of an interpretive phenomenological methodology refer to Chapters 3 and 12.)

Interpretive phenomenology's central project is 'to generate converging conversations from cycles in the hermeneutic circle of interpreting, understanding and critiquing texts' (Darbyshire *et al.* 1999, p. 18). Heidegger viewed phenomenology as 'destruction', which means 'looking past the normal, everyday meanings of life to see the larger meaning of Being' (Cohen and Omery 1994, p. 141). The hermeneutic-phenomenological view is therefore ontologic in approach (Ray 1994).

However, before the advent of Martin Heidegger, Max Scheler 'was in the eyes of the German public the number two phenomenologist' and 'he probably did more for the spread of the entire [phenomenological] movement abroad, especially in the French- and Spanish-speaking world, than any other phenomenologist' (Spiegelberg 1971/1965, p. 228).

Existential phenomenology

Heidegger, 'the second intellectual pillar in phenomenology' (Gearing 2004, p. 1431), is accredited with giving phenomenology an 'existentialist' orientation. However, Crotty (1996) argues that Heidegger 'forthrightly rejected the existential tag' and in 1946 openly denounced an association with the existentialist views of Sarte (p. 65). Existential phenomenology applies phenomenology to human existence because of its view that existence can be studied the same as other phenomenon and its essential structures uncovered (Hein and Austin 2001). Existential phenomenologists in their advancement of phenomenology, emphasized the lifeworld (Ashworth 2008). Existential phenomenology emphasizes 'embodiment (we are in the world as bodies) and our dynamic relationship with the world (we act upon the world and, in turn, are acted upon)' (Crotty 1996, p. 68). Intentionality, when viewed with an existentialist lens 'ceases to be expressed in purely epistemological terms. It becomes ontological... existential phenomenologists describe human being itself as intentionally orientated towards space and time' (Crotty 1996, p. 40). Moreover,

Heidegger does not include Husserl's position on natural attitude, *epoché,* or reduction in his work *Being in Time* (Moran 2000).

Heidegger's work steered away from a study of essences and rather he viewed interpretation as a core aspect of our *being-in-the-world* (Gearing 2004). He developed existential and hermeneutic aspects of phenomenology and directed focus on the historical/cultural contexts of the phenomenologi-cal project (Finlay 2008). Heidegger therefore argued that presuppositions should not be 'eliminated or suspended, but are what constitute the possibil-ity of intelligibility or meaning' (Ray 1994, p. 120). Moreover, Heidegger's view of phenomenology suggests that many interpretations can be revealed, whereas Husserl's view regards only one interpretation from the data (Hein and Austin 2001).

Heidegger 'has unquestionably the largest following' (Spiegelberg 1971/1965, p. 353). Heidegger was influenced by the Danish philosopher Soren Kierkegaard (1813–1955), regarded as the founder of existential philos-ophy (Valle *et al.* 1989) and was one of the first to combine existential thinking with phenomenological methodology. Heidegger considered that his work, *Being in Time,* published in 1927 after 20 years of a 'never-ending search for the meaning of being' was misunderstood (Crotty 1996, p. 65). Nevertheless, Heidegger's work of combining existential and phenomenology thinking attracted international attention from many, including the young minds of Sarte, Merleau-Ponty, Arendt, Macuse and many others (Kearney 1994).

Sarte went to Berlin in 1933 for nine months to study the phenome-nology of Husserl, Scheler, Jaspers and Heidegger (Crotty 1996). In 1946, Sarte's popular work on phenomenology *Existentialismand Humanism* was published (Kearney 1994). Sarte believed that his humanistic brand of phenomenological existentialism provided 'a radically new beginning' to 'a population disillusioned with traditional systems of meaning' at the end of the war (Kearney 1994, pp. 52–53). He later encouraged Merleau-Ponty to read Husserl's *Ideas,* and this resulted in Sarte and Merleau-Ponty lead-ing the existential phenomenology movement (Crotty 1996). In order for all this to have occurred, credit must be given to Fink who, along with a young German priest, Herman Leo Van Breda, smuggled Husserl's manu-scripts out of Nazi Germany to the Catholic University of Leuven (Moran 2007). On 1 April 1939, Merleau-Ponty was the first visitor to Leuven to read Husserl's typescripts (Moran 2007), and the rest, so to speak, is history.

The interpretive approach outlined by Diekelmann *et al.* (1989) is based on Heideggerian phenomenology. The focus of Diekelmann *et al.*'s approach is to uncover 'taken for granted shared practices and common meanings' (Cohen and Omery 1994, p. 150). This approach is labelled as a 'third tradition' in phenomenology; the other two being Dutch phenom-enology (discussed later in this chapter) and the Duquesne tradition of phenomenology (referred to earlier) (Cohen and Omery 1994). The inter-pretive approach based on Heideggerian phenomenology remains popular. For instance, Adolfsson *et al.* (2004) utilized interpretive phenomenology based on the work of Heidegger 'to identify and describe women's experience of miscarriage'. Also, using an interpretive phenomenological approach influenced by Heidegger, Siwe *et al.* (2006) describe the experience of being a professional patient in teaching the pelvic examination to medical and midwifery students.

Hermeneutics

Research methodologies based on Heidegger's writings are not only considered interpretive but also hermeneutic (Draucker 1999). Heidegger also built on the work of Schleiermacher (1768–1834) and Dilthey (1833–1911) on hermeneutics. Unlike descriptive/Husserlian phenomenology discussed earlier, hermeneutic phenomenology is a philosophy that aims to achieve understanding through interpretation and adopts a process that clarifies the phenomenon of interest in its context as opposed to presenting its essential structure (Hein and Austin 2001).

The term 'hermeneutics' originated in the seventeenth century to describe a method used for biblical and classical literary interpretation to illuminate the meaning of the text (Eberhart and Pieper 1994). In more recent times, hermeneutics has moved from being regarded as a secondary aspect of European philosophy to being one of the most extensively debated topics in contemporary philosophy (Bowie 1998).

Hermeneutics as a research method is based on the belief that 'lived experience itself is essentially an interpretive process' (Cohen and Omery 1994, p. 148). Also of importance to highlight is that with a hermeneutic approach, questioning of research participants can adopt a conceptual, theoretical or historical stance (Ray 1994). This approach to questioning is very different from that adopted with descriptive phenomenology. The result of a hermeneutic phenomenological approach 'is a piece of writing that explicates the meaning of human phenomena and helps to understand the lived structures of meaning' (Ehrich 2005, p. 5).

Gadamer (1990) and Ricoeur (1981) subsequently further developed ideas on a hermeneutic phenomenology. Hans-Georg Gadamer is accredited with developing what we know as 'phenomenological hermeneutics'. Gadamer (2004) contests that elimination of individual prejudices is not only impossible it is also unnecessary. He supports this argument by stating that its absence can interfere with the interpretation process. The sociohistory and culture of the researcher with this strand of hermeneutics is considered 'an essential part of the interpreter's development of understanding and therefore critical to the research process' (Doyle 2007, p. 888). Gadamer (1990) used the metaphor 'fusion of horizons' and proposed that understanding will evolve following a fusion of horizons between the researcher and participant. However, because a current horizon is constantly evolving, a new understanding between researcher and participant must become one understanding (Fleming *et al.* 2003).

Gadamer (1990) also talks about the lifeworld. According to Gadamer (1990) the lifeworld can be accessed through 'openness'. Openness is inextricably linked to the notion of the 'phenomenological attitude'. Being open means approaching phenomena as they appear and in doing so suspending presuppositions (Dahlberg *et al.* 2001).

Fleming *et al.* (2003) propose a five-step process to be adopted when undertaking phenomenogical research guided by Gadamer's view of hermeneutics. Furthermore, Crist and Tanner (2003) outline methods that researchers can adopt in interpretation and analysis with hermeneutic interpretive phenomenology. The interpretive hermeneutic approach to phenomenology is popular. For instance, using a hermeneutic approach guided by the writings of Heidegger and Gadamer, Thomson and Downe (2008) explored the lived experience and personal meanings attached to a traumatic birth. (Also refer to Chapters 5, 6, 8, 10 and 12 for research utilizing an interpretive/hermeneutic approach.)

Of interest is the utilization of Colaizzi's approach (from the Duquesne school) in some phenomenological studies described as interpretive. For instance, Harris *et al.* (2003) utilize Colaizzi's (1978) approach in their hermeneutical study of women's perspective of breasts and breastfeeding in the early month after birthing. Colaizzi's final step in his method involves the researcher returning to participants and asking how the researcher's descriptive results compare with the participants' experiences. This suggests some interpretation is acknowledged, rather than just description.

Ricoeur's role in hermeneutic phenomenology

The work of French philosopher, Paul Ricoeur also deserves mention. Ricoeur, influenced by Heidegger and Gadamer, took his work on phenomenology beyond 'eidetic' and 'existentialist' phenomenology towards a phenomenology that was 'hermeneutic' in its focus (Kearney 1994), and is viewed to have offered the 'broadest' view of phenomenology and hermeneutics (Ray 1994, p. 121).

Ricoeur 'attempted to reconcile the presuppositionless and interpretive phenomenologic gulf of Husserlian and Heideggerian methodology' (Ray 1994, p. 129). He rejected Husserl's view on the suspension of presuppositions (Kearney 1994), and argued that phenomenology should go further than mere description of experience towards interpretation (Ricoeur 1981).

Ricoeur's work has influenced the development of a branch of phenomenology known as the Vancouver School of phenomenology (Halldorsdottir 2000). This is described as 'an interpretation of phenomenological constructivist/interpretivist philosophy' and 'a unique blend of description, interpretation, explication and construction' (Halldorsdottir 2000, p. 53), which is also influenced by Spiegelberg's work on phenomenology and Swandt's work on constructivism. The Vancouver method has been utilized in a number of studies with a nursing and midwifery focus, including a study by Halldorsdottir and Karlsdottir (1996) which explored women's experiences of labour and delivery.

Similar to the approach mentioned earlier by Pollio *et al.* (1997), the Vancouver School of phenomenology also outlines a series of steps to guide researchers. The Vancouver School has 12 steps: sample selection, silence, data collection, data analysis, coding, individual case construction, verification of single case construction with the study participants (co-researchers), meta-synthesis of all the case constructions, comparison of the essential structure with the data, interpreting the meaning of the phenomenon, verifying the findings with some of the study participants, and writing up the findings (Halldorsdottir 2000). The second stage is labelled 'first, there is silence', the goal of which is that the researcher 'opens-up, sharpens his or her receptive faculties and is ready to hear something new' (Halldorsdottir 2000, p. 59). During this phase, the researcher should read as much as possible on the phenomenon under scrutiny 'in an attempt to become free from narrow preconstruction of the phenomenon' (Halldorsdotir 2000, p. 59). This differs from the advice to researchers adopting descriptive phenomenology not to undertake a literature review prior the data collection (Streubert and Carpenter 1999). The Vancouver method is also compared to its similarities with grounded theory (Peturrson 2005). However, unlike grounded theory, with the Vancouver method 'participants have a more active role…and therefore can break the interviewer's monopoly of interpretation' (Petursson 2005, p. 121).

Van Manen's approach

Habermas and others in North America have also made contributions to the contemporary developments in phenomenology and hermeneutics (Ray 1994). Van Manen was influenced by the Utrecht school, or the German phenomenological tradition, and hermeneutic phenomenological philosophy (Ehrich 2005), and he emphasizes the importance of writing in his research method (Smith *et al.* 2009). This approach is labelled Dutch phenomenology of the 'Utrecht school'. Martinus Langeveld (1905–1989) was a key founder of the Utrecht school in The Netherlands. Kockelmans (1987) also belongs to this group.

Van Manen (2006) argues that the practice of writing cannot be divorced from phenomenological enquiry. He also warns of the dangers of phenomenological method and urges phenomenological researchers to 'resist the temptation to surrender to a view of method that hollows out our understandings and cuts us off from the deeper sources of meaning' (van Manen 2006, p. 714). Nevertheless, similar to that of empirical phenomenology, he does endorse the role of imaginative free variation in pursuit of a phenomenon's essence (Ehrich 2005).

Van Manen's approach is popular. For instance, Lundqvist *et al.* (2002) drew inspiration from van Manen (1997) during interviewing and analysis in their study that described mothers' experience of professional care when their newborn dies. Also, van Manen's (1990) principles of hermeneutic phenomenology are utilized by Ross *et al.* (2007) in a study which describes the lived experience of HIV-positive pregnant women in Thailand. Finally, his approach is utilized by Berg and Honkasalo (2000) in their hermeneutic phenomenological study which interviewed pregnant women with diabetes.

Benner (1994) is accredited with introducing interpretive phenomenology based on Heideggerian phenomenology into nursing circles (Draucker 1999). Benner's (1994) approach to phenomenology (interpretive phenomenology) draws heavily on the work of Heidegger and is considered similar to the approach of van Manen (Smith *et al.* 2009). Benner's (1984) use of 'exemplars' or 'paradigm cases' are highlighted by Ray (1994) as suitable to capture a 'transformative experience' (p. 128) such as pregnancy. A number of studies have utilized Benner's (1994) interpretive phenomenological approach within the childbirth and maternity care arena. For example Cibulka (2007) explored pregnancy intention and conception practices of HIV-infected women. Su and Chen (2006) studied the lived experience of infertile women who terminated treatment after *in vitro* fertilization failure. In addition, Sweet and Darbyshire (2007) utilize Benner's approach to uncover fathers' views of breastfeeding of their preterm baby.

Van Manen's approach is considered one of a 'family of approaches, a fuzzy set where all share the basic tenets of phenomenology but each articulates an approach in a particular way' (Smith *et al.* 2009, p. 200). Another member of that family is a recent approach in psychology informed by Ricoeur labelled 'critical narrative analysis' (Langdridge 2008). Also gaining interest is the dialogical approach to phenomenology (Halling *et al.* 1994).

Criticisms of North American phenomenology

Crotty (1996) labels descriptive phenomenology in North American developments 'new phenomenology' (p. 2). Criticism from Crotty (1996) and Paley (1997) of 'new phenomenology' has placed a spotlight on phenomenological research. Crotty (1996) argued that 'the fruit it [new phenomenology] has produced reflects the American intellectual tradition far more than any features of the parent [European phenomenology] plant' (p. 2). In addition, he argues that new phenomenology misinterprets intentionality because it is concerned mostly with the subjective and is 'not based on the bringing together of objectivity and subjectivity which intentionality encapsulates' (Crotty 1996, p. 42). Lawler (1998) raises a similar point and reminds readers that a 'different kind of phenomenology' (p. 106) has evolved in the USA, where 'the intellectual climate…typifies their cultural and social mores and history' (p. 106). Lawler's (1998) excellent paper also argues that 'one cannot "be" in a culture-free way' (p. 107).

However, phenomenology is 'a moving, in contrast to a stationary philosophy, with a dynamic momentum' (Spiegelberg 1971/1965, p. 2). Moreover, Natanson (1973) argues that 'philosophy provides a fundamental perspective in terms of which the pieces of the work of the social scientist can be put together in a coherent unity' (p. 31). Similarly, as discussed earlier, Polkinghorne (1989) and Giorgi (2000a,b) both argue explicitly that phenomenology as a philosophy is distinct from phenomenology as a scientific practice. Moreover, Giorgi argues that if researchers were to pursue the philosophy of Husserl as it was originally conceived, they would be practising philosophy, rather than research (Giorgi 2000a,b).

Discussion and conclusion

The variety of approaches to phenomenology available to researchers are many, with various labels attached (Table 4.1).

Table 4.1 Summary of types of phenomenological approaches and key promoters

Phenomenological approaches	*Key promoters*
Descriptive phenomenology	• van Kaam (1959, 1966) [Duquesne School] [USA] • Colaizzi (1978) [Duquesne School] [USA] • Giorgi [Duquesne School] (1985, 1986, 1994, 1997, 2000a,b, 2005, 2008) [USA] • Polkinghorne (1989) [USA] • Moustakas (1994) [USA] • Pollio's approach to existential-phenomenology (Pollio *et al.* 1997) [USA] • Dallas Approach (Garza 2007) [influenced by Duquesne school] [USA]
Lifeworld phenomenology	• Dahlberg and Todres (Dahlberg *et al.* 2001, Todres *et al.* 2007) [Sweden] • Ashworth (2003) [England]
Interpretive phenomenology	• Diekelmann *et al.* (1989) [Heidegger] [USA] • Benner (1994) [Heidegger] [USA]
Hermeneutic phenomenology	• Fleming *et al.* (2003) [Gadamer] [Scotland] • Vancouver school (Halldorsdottir 2000) [Ricoeur] [Canada]
Mixture of descriptive, interpretive and hermeneutic	• van Manen (1990) [Canada] • Interpretative Phenomenological Analysis (IPA) Smith *et al.* (2009) [England]

The driving force of psychology on the development of phenomenological approaches is evident in the many approaches from the USA, principally driven by those of the Duquesne school. In the UK, psychology's influence is also evident in developments in IPA and lifeworld phenomenology from Sheffield University (Ashworth 2003). The influence of nursing and midwifery is evident in the interpretive and hermeneutic approaches developed by Diekelmann *et al.* (1989), Benner (1994), Fleming *et al.* (2003) and work from the Vancouver school (Halldorsdottir 2000), and lifeworld phenomenology (Dahlberg *et al.* 2001, Todres *et al.* 2007).

This diversity of approaches requires researchers to be cognisant of the philosophical underpinnings directing their choice. Undertaking phenomenological research without this philosophical understanding puts the integrity of the research study at risk. Differentiating interpretive and hermeneutic phenomenology from descriptive phenomenology is essential to this understanding. The phenomenological method promoted by those who follow the school of descriptive phenomenology utilized in phenomenological psychology is best summarized by Merleau-Ponty under four key characteristics as follows: it is descriptive, it utilizes reduction, it searches for essences and it is focused on intentionality (De Castro 2003). This approach emphasizes the importance of a rigorous process when undertaking data analysis. However, the focus of interpretive/hermeneutic phenomenology is on interpreting and understanding with intentionality viewed with an existentialist lens, rendering it ontological in perspective (Crotty 2006).

Smith *et al.* (2009) argue that although the focus of various phenomenologists differs, they all are generally interested in what it is to be human and what constitutes our lived world. Moreover, all types of phenomenological research approaches utilize one or more sources of data (the researcher's reflections pertaining to the phenomenon under investigation, the participants' verbal or written accounts of the phenomenon and descriptions of the phenomenon assembled from literature, media and other phenomenological research) (Hein and Austin 2001). What needs to be emphasized is that there is no 'one way' of undertaking a phenomenological study. The choice of approach depends on many issues, such as the nature of the research question, the data collected, and the aim of the researcher as well as their abilities (Hein and Austin 2001). This latter advice from Hein and Austin (2001) is one that I often use when discussing with students and colleagues which phenomenological approach is the most appropriate for their particular study. I encourage anyone who is embarking on a phenomenological study to firstly consider their own aim for their study and where they see themselves in their study.

My own personal view on phenomenological research approaches has evolved over several years of reading and undertaking a variety of studies utilizing various perspectives. Where I stand now is very different to the viewpoint I took a decade ago. I am currently particularly drawn to the Vancouver School (Halldorsdottir 2000) of phenomenology and Pollio *et al*'s (1997) approach. Pollio *et al.* (1997) encourage the researcher to focus on the self initially. This involves the researcher being interviewed by a member of the interpretive team before the study begins. The researcher and the interpretive team then interpret the interview text, in order to uncover the researcher's views on the topic. Furthermore, the interpretive group support the researcher throughout the study and offer 'competing perspectives' (Secrest 2007, p. 5). Similar to Pollio *et al*'s approach, Halldorsdottir (2000) encourages the researcher to embrace a 'silence' so that the researcher 'opens up, sharpens his or her receptive faculties and is ready to hear something new' (p. 59). Although these two approaches belong to different phenomenological perspectives (see Table 4.1), the initial focus on the self is common to them both and I believe this focus sets the appropriate tone for a study as a whole. In addition, Pollio *et al.*'s (1997) approach and the Vancouver School (Halldorsdottir 2000) outline an explicit process, which guides the research study. Novice researchers to phenomenology in particular will find such a process useful guidance. I also find myself drawn to the writings of Finlay (2006, 2008, 2009), who eloquently captures the essence of the phenomenological researcher's 'sense of wonder and openness to the world' (Finlay 2008, p. 2), and has helped me appreciate phenomenological reduction from a deeper perspective.

It is appropriate therefore to conclude this chapter by referring to Finlay (2009), who asks the important question of what counts as phenomenology. She goes further and answers her own question with emphasis on the researcher also, with the assertion that 'phenomenological research is phenomenological when it involves both rich description of the lifeworld or lived experience, and where the researcher has adopted a special, open phenomenological attitude' (Finlay 2009, p. 8). Finlay's (2009) view encompasses the many varieties of phenomenology, and there is no doubt of the popularity of this research approach. However, Lawler (1998) expresses concern that the popularity of phenomenology and its many varieties may put it at risk of becoming a 'boutique methodology' (p. 108). However, like Garza (2007), I take the view that 'the adaptability of [phenomenology's] methods to ever widening arcs of enquiry is one of its greatest strengths' (p. 338).

References

Adolfsson A., Larsson P.G., Wijma B. and Bertero C. (2004) Guilt and emptiness: Women's experiences of miscarriage. *Health Care for Women International* 25, 543–560.

Ashworth P. (1996) Presuppose nothing! The suspension of assumptions in phenomenological psychological methodology. *Journal of Phenomenological Psychology* 27, 1–25.

Ashworth P. (2003) An approach to phenomenological psychology: the contingencies of the lifeworld. *Journal of Phenomenological Psychology* 34, 145–156.

Ashworth P. (2008) Conceptual foundations of qualitative psychology. In *Qualitative Psychology: A Practical Guide for Research Methods* (Smith J.A. ed.) (2nd edn). Sage: London: 4–25.

Benner P. (1984) *From Novice to Expert: Excellence and Power in Clinical Nursing Practice.* Addison-Wesley: Reading, MA.

Benner P. (1994) The tradition and skill in interpretive phenomenology in studying health, illness and caring practices. In *Interpretive Phenomenology* (Benner P. ed.) Sage: Thousand Oaks, California: 99–128.

Berg M. and Honkasalo M.L. (2000) Pregnancy and diabetes – A hermeneutic phenomenological study of women's experiences. *Journal of Psychosomatic Obstetrics and Gynaecology* 21, 39–48.

Berndtsson I., Claesson S., Friberg F. and Öhlén J. (2007) Issues about thinking phenomenologically while doing phenomenology. *Journal of Phenomenological Psychology* 38, 256–277.

Biley F.C. and Galvin K.T. (2007) Lifeworld, the arts and mental health nursing. *Journal of Psychiatric and Mental Health Nursing* 14, 800–807.

Bleicher J. (1980) *Contemporary Hermeneutics.* Routledge & Kegan Paul: London.

Bowie A. (1998) (ed.) *Schleiermacher. Hermeneutics and Criticism.* Cambridge University Press: Cambridge.

Cerbone D.R. (2006) *Understanding Phenomenology.* Acumen: Chesham, Bucks.

Chang S.N. and Mu P.F. (2008) Infertile couples' experience of family stress while women are hospitalized for Ovarian Hyperstimulation Syndrome during infertility treatment. *Journal of Clinical Nursing* 17, 531–538.

Cibulka N.J. (2007) Conception Practices of HIV-Infected Women in the Midwest. *Journal of the Association of Nurses in AIDS Care* 18, 3–12.

Clemmens D.A. (2002) Adolescent mothers' depression after the birth of their babies: Weathering the storm. *Adolescence* 37, 550–565.

Cohen M.Z. and Omery A. (1994) Schools of phenomenology: implications for research. In *Critical Issues in Qualitative Research Methods.* (Morse J.M. ed). Sage: Thousand Oaks, California: 136–156.

Costelloe T.M. (1996) Between the subject and sociology: Alfred Schutz's phenomenology of the lifeworld. *Human Studies* 19, 247–266.

Colaizzi P.E. (1978) Psychological research as the phenomenologist views it. In *Existential–Phenomenological Alternatives for Psychology.* (Valle R.S. and King M. eds), Oxford University Press: New York: 48–71.

Crist J.D. and Tanner C.A. (2003) Interpretation/analysis methods in hermeneutic interpretive phenomenology. *Nursing research,* 52, 202–205.

Crotty M. (1996) *Phenomenology and Nursing Research.* Churchill Livingstone: Melbourne.

Dahlberg K.M.E. and Dahlberg H.K. (2004) Description vs. interpretation – a new understanding of an old dilemma in human science research. *Nursing Philosophy* 5, 268–273.

Dahlberg K., Dahlberg H. and Nystrom M. (2001) (eds) *Reflective lifeworld research.* Studentlitteratur: Lund, Sweden.

Darbyshire P., Diekelmann J. and Diekelmann N. (1999) Reading Heidegger and interpretive phenomenology: A response to the work of Michael Crotty. *Nursing Inquiry* 6, 17–25.

De Castro A. (2003) Introduction to Giorgi's existential phenomenological research method. *Psichologia Desde El Caribe. Universidad Del Norte* 11, 45–56.

Diekelmann, N. (2001) Preface. In, Dahlberg K., Dahlberg H. and Nystrom M. (2001) (eds) *Reflective lifeworld research.* Studentlitteratur: Lund, Sweden.

Diekelmann N., Allen D. and Tanner C. (1989) *The NLN Criteria for Appraisal of Baccalaureate Programs: A Critical Hermeneutic Analysis.* National League for Nursing Press: New York.

Doyle S. (2007) Member checking with older women: A framework for negotiating meaning. *Health Care for Women International* 28, 888–908.

Draucker C.B. (1999) The critique of Heideggerian hermeneutical nursing research. *Journal of Advanced Nursing* 30, 360–373.

Eberhart C. and Pieper B.B. (1994) Understanding Human action through narrative expression and Hermeneutic inquiry. In *Advances in Methods of Inquiry for Nursing* (Chinn P. ed), Aspen publications: Maryland: 41–58.

Ehrich L. (2005) Revisiting phenomenology: its potential for management research. In *Proceedings challenges or organisations in global markets,* British Academy of Management conference, Said University School: Oxford University: 1–13.

Embree L. (2008) The nature and role of phenomenological psychology in Alfred Schutz. *Journal of Phenomenological Psychology* 39, 141–150.

Finlay L. (2006) The body's disclosure in phenomenological research. *Qualitative Research in Psychology* 3, 19–30.

Finlay L. (2008) A dance between the reduction and reflexivity: Explicating the 'phenomenological psychological attitude'. *Journal of Phenomenological Psychology* 39, 1–32.

Finlay L. (2009) Debating phenomenological research methods. *Phenomenology and Practice* 3, 6–25.

Fleming V., Gaidys U. and Robb Y. (2003) Hermeneutic research in nursing: developing a Gadamerian-based research method. *Nursing Inquiry* 10, 113–120.

Gadamer H.G. (1990) *Truth and Method.* (Weinsheimer J. and Marshall D. trans.) (2nd rev. edn) Crossroad: New York.

Gadamer H.G. (2004) *Truth and Method.* (3rd rev. Edn) Continuum: London.

Garza G. (2007) Varieties of phenomenological research at the University of Dallas: An emerging typology. *Qualitative Research in Psychology* 4, 313–342.

Gearing R.E. (2004) Bracketing in research: A typology. *Qualitative Health Research* 14, 1429–1452.

Giorgi A. (1985) The phenomenological psychology of learning and the verbal learning tradition. In *Phenomenology and Psychological Research* (Giorgi A. ed.) Duquesne University Press: Pittsburgh, PA: 23–85.

Giorgi, A. (1986) *A Phenomenological Analysis of Descriptions of Conceptions of Learning Obtained from a Phenomenographic Perspective.* Department of Education: Göteborg University.

Giorgi A. (1994) A phenomenological perspective on certain qualitative research methods. *Journal of Phenomenological Psychology* 25, 190–220.

Giorgi A. (1997) The theory, practice and the evaluation of the phenomenological method as a qualitative research procedure. *Journal of Phenomenological Psychology* 28, 235–260.

Giorgi A. (2000a) The status of Husserlian Phenomenology in caring research. *Scandinavian Journal of Caring Science* 14, 3–10.

Giorgi A. (2000b) Concerning the application of phenomenology to caring research. *Scandinavian Journal of Caring Science* 14, 11–15.

Giorgi A. (2005) The phenomenological movement and research in the human sciences. *Nursing Science Quarterly* 18, 75–82.

Giorgi A. (2008) Concerning a serious misunderstanding of the essence of the phenomenological method in psychology. *Journal of Phenomenological Psychology* 39, 33–58.

Greenwood D. and Lowenthal D. (2005) Case study as a means of researching social work and improving practitioner education. *Journal of Social Work Practice* 19, 181–193.

Halldorsdottir S. (2000) The Vancouver School of doing phenomenology. In *Qualitative Methods in Service of Health* (Fridlund B. and Hildingh C. eds) Studentlitteratur: Lund, Sweden: 47–81.

Halldorsdottir S. and Karlsdottir S.I. (1996) Journeying through labour and delivery: Perceptions of women who have given birth. *Midwifery* 12, 48–61.

Halling S., Kunz G. and Rowe J.O. (1994) The contributions of dialogal psychology to phenomenological research. *Journal of Humanistic Psychology* 34, 1.

Harris M., Nayda R. and Summers A. (2003) Breasts and breastfeeding: perspectives of women in the early months after birthing. *Breastfeeding Review* 11, 21–29.

Hein S.F. and Austin W.J. (2001) Empirical and hermeneutic approaches to phenomenological research in psychology: A comparison. *Psychological Methods* 6, 3–17.

Hunter L.P. (2008) A hermeneutic phenomenological analysis of midwives' ways of knowing during childbirth. *Midwifery* 24, 405–415.

Husserl E. (1970/1936) *The Crisis of European Sciences and Transcendental Phenomenology: An Introduction to Phenomenological Philosophy.* Northwestern University Press (Original work published 1936).

Johansson M. and Berg M. (2005) Women's experiences of childlessness 2 years after the end of in vitro fertilization treatment. *Scandinavian Journal of Caring Sciences* 19, 58–63.

Kearney R. (1994) *Modern Movements in European Philosophy.* (2nd edn), Manchester University Press: Manchester.

Kockelmans J.J. (ed.) (1987) *Phenomenological Psychology: The Dutch School.* Martinus Nijhoff Publishers: Dordrecht, The Netherlands.

Langdridge D. (2008) Phenomenology and critical social psychology: Directions and debates in theory and research. *Social and Personality Psychology Compass* 2, 1126–1142.

Lawler J. (1998) Phenomenologies as research methodologies for nursing: From philosophy to researching practice. *Nursing Inquiry* 5, 104–111.

LeVasseur J.J. (2003) The problem of bracketing in phenomenology. *Qualitative Health Research* 13, 408–420.

Lowes L. and Prowse M.A. (2001) Standing outside the interview process? The illusion of objectivity in phenomenological data generation. *International Journal of Nursing Studies* 38, 471–480.

Lundqvist A., Nilstun T. and Dykes A.K. (2002) Both empowered and powerless: Mothers' experiences of professional care when their newborn dies. *Birth* 29, 192–199.

Lundgren I. and Dahlberg K. (2002) Midwives' experience of the encounter with women and their pain during childbirth. *Midwifery* 18, 155–164.

McNamara M.S. (2005) Knowing and doing phenomenology: The implications of the critique of 'nursing phenomenology' for a phenomenological inquiry: A discussion paper. *International Journal of Nursing Studies* 42, 695–704.

Meighan M., Davis M.W., Thomas S.P. and Droppleman P.G. (1999) Living with postpartum depression: The father's experience. *MCN The American Journal of Maternal Child Nursing* 24, 202–208.

Merleau-Ponty M. (1962) *The Phenomenology of Perception.* (Smith C. trans). Humanities Press: New York.

Moran D. (2000) *Introduction to Phenomenology.* Routledge: London.

Moran D. (2007) Fink's speculative phenomenology: Between constitution and transcendence. *Research in Phenomenology* 37, 3–31.

Moustakas C. (1994) *Phenomenological Research Methods,* Sage: Thousand Oaks, California.

Natanson M. (ed.) (1973) *Phenomenology and the Social Sciences, Volume 1.* Northwestern University Press: Evanston.

Owen I.R. (1994) Introducing an existential-phenomenological approach: basic phenomenological theory and research – Part 1. *Psychology Quarterly* 7, 261–274.

Paley J. (1997) Husserl, phenomenology and nursing. *Journal of Advanced Nursing* 26, 187–193.

Peterson W.E., Sword W., Charles C. and DiCenso A. (2007) Adolescents' perceptions of inpatient postpartum nursing care. *Qualitative Health Research* 17, 201–212.

Petursson P. (2005) GPs' reasons for 'non-pharmacological' prescribing of antibiotics: A phenomenological study. *Scandinavian Journal of Primary Health Care* 23, 120–125.

Polkinghorne D. (1989) Phenomenological research methods. In *Existential– Phenomenological Perspectives in Psychology* (Valle R. and Halling S. eds) Plenum: New York: 41–60.

Pollio H.R., Thompson C.B. and Henley, T. (1997) *The Phenomenology of Everyday Life.* Cambridge University Press: Cambridge.

Ray M.A. (1994) The richness of phenomenology: Philosophic, Theoretic, and Methodologic Concerns. In *Critical Issues in Qualitative Research Method,* (Morse, J.M. ed.) Sage: Thousand Oaks, California: 116–133.

Ricoeur P. (1981) *Hermeneutics and the Human Sciences,* (J. Thompson ed. and trans.) Cambridge University Press: New York.

Ricoeur P. (1967) *Husserl. An Analysis of his Phenomenology.* Northwestern University Press: Illinois.

Rolls L. and Relf. M (2004) 'Bracketing interviews': a method for increasing objectivity in bereavement and palliative care research. Paper presented at *Methodology of Research in Palliative care.* Third research forum of the EAPC, June: Stresa, Italy.

Ross R., Sawatphanit W., Draucker C.B. and Suwansujarid T. (2007) The lived experiences of HIV-positive, pregnant women in Thailand. *Health Care for Women International* 28, 731–744.

Secrest J.A. (2007) Pollio's approach to existential phenomenology: a brief synopsis. *Journal of PeriAnesthesia Nursing* 22, 5–9.

Siwe K., Wijma B. and Berterö C. (2006) 'A stronger and clearer perception of self'. Women's experience of being professional patients in teaching the pelvic examination: A qualitative study. *BJOG: An International Journal of Obstetrics and Gynaecology* 113, 890–895.

Smith J.A., Flowers P. and Larkin M. (2009) *Interpretative Phenomenological Analysis: Theory, Method and Research.* Sage: London.

Spiegelberg H. (1971/1965) *The Phenomenological Movement: A Historical Introduction* (2nd edn) Martinus Nijhoff: The Hague.

Spiegelberg H. (1982/1965) *The Phenomenological Movement: A Historical Introduction.* Martinus Nijhoff: The Hague.

Streubert H.J. and Carpenter D.R. (1999) *Qualitative Research in Nursing: Advancing the Humanistic Imperative.* Lippincott: New York.

Su T.J. and Chen Y.C. (2006) Transforming hope: the lived experience of infertile women who terminated treatment after in vitro fertilization failure. *The Journal of Nursing Research* 14, 46–54.

Sweet L. and Darbyshire P. (2007) Fathers and breastfeeding very-low-birthweight preterm babies. *Midwifery* 25, 540–553.

Thomson G. and Downe S. (2008) Widening the trauma discourse: The link between childbirth and experiences of abuse. *Journal of Psychosomatic Obstetrics and Gynecology* 29, 268–273.

Thomas S.P. (2005) Through the lens of Merleau-Ponty: advancing the phenomenological approach to nursing research. *Nursing Philosophy* 6, 63–76.

Todres L., Galvin K. and Dahlberg K. (2007) Lifeworld-led healthcare: Revisiting a humanising philosophy that integrates emerging trends. *Medicine, Healthcare and Philosophy* 10, 53–63.

Valle R.S., King M. and Halling S. (1989) An introduction to Existential-Phenomenological thought in Psychology, In *Existential–Phenomenological Perspectives in Psychology: Exploring the Breadth of Human Experience.* (Valle R.S. and Halling S. eds) Plenum Press: New York: 3–16.

van Kaam A. (1959) Phenomenal analysis: Exemplified by a study of the experience of 'really feeling understood'. *Journal of Individual Psychology* 15, 66–72.

van Kaam A. (1966) *Existential foundations of psychology.* Duquesne University Press: Pittsburgh, PA.

van Manen M. (1990) *Researching Lived Experience: Human Science for an Action Sensitive Pedagogy.* Althouse Press: Ontario.

van Manen M. (1997) *Researching Lived Experience: Human Science for an Action Sensitive Pedagogy* (2nd edn). Althouse Press: Ontario.

van Manen M. (2006) Writing qualitatively or the demands of writing. *Qualitative Health Research* 16(5): 713–722.

Wagner H.R. (1970) Introduction. In *On phenomenology and social relations* (Schutz, A., ed.) Chicago University Press: Chicago: 1–52.

Wilson T.D. (2002) Alfred Scutz, phenomenology and research methodology for information behaviour research. Paper delivered at *ISIC4 – Fourth International Conference on Information Seeking in Context,* Universidade Lusiada: Lisbon, Portugal: September 11 to 13, 2002.

Zaner R.M. and Ihde D. (1973) *Phenomenology and Existentialism.* Capricorn Books, GP Putman's Sons: New York.

5 Lesbian women's experiences of being different in Irish health care

Mel Duffy

Introduction

This chapter focuses upon lesbian women's experiences of 'being different' in Irish health care, whether that is being made to feel different or knowing one's difference, regardless of interaction with others. Heidegger (1962, p. 63) suggests, '[T]his thing that is called difference, we encounter it everywhere'. Research suggests that lesbian women experience their difference in health care through societal views, of what is 'normal', and 'natural' sexuality (Taylor 1999); assumptions of heterosexuality (Lehmann *et al.* 1998); and the specific health care needs of lesbian women (Marrazzo *et al.* 2005). This chapter presents five lesbian women's experiences of being lesbian in Irish health care from a hermeneutical phenomenological perspective. A description of the theoretical and methodological approach adopted for this study is provided. Implications for practice are also discussed.

Being lesbian in Irish society

> It is in the reality of everyday life that the 'Other' appears to us, and his probability refers to everyday reality.
>
> (Sartre 1969, p. 253)

There is limited knowledge about lesbian women's lives and social experiences in Irish society. Research suggests that lesbian women are indistinguishable within the social structures and institutions of society (Lemon and Patton 1997), which include education (Norman *et al.* 2006), religion (Kenny 1997) and family (Hug 1999). However, there has been a change in Irish public attitudes towards lesbian women and gay men, with 53 per cent indicating that sex between same-sex couples was 'never wrong' (Layte *et al.* 2006). Layte *et al.* (2006) suggest that the history of stigmatization of homosexuality in Irish society may distort these figures as 'all estimates of same-sex attraction, experience and identity based upon self-report should be seen as under-estimates' (Layte *et al.* 2006, p. 127). This would suggest that some lesbian and gay men in Irish society may feel uncomfortable in identifying their sexuality in a confidential questionnaire.

In the last 20 years Irish society has experienced significant legislative changes, reflected in the decriminalization of homosexuality in 1993, the Employment Equality Act, 1997 and the Equal Status Act, 2000; all of which should have led to an ease of living for lesbian women in Irish society. However, it is argued that social attitudes take longer to come in line with the law, particularly in relation to sexuality:

> Sexual orientation, identity and expression do not occur in a neutral environment where sexual identity ... is a simple matter of individual choice. Quite the opposite; homosexuality is still widely stigmatized and homosexual identity can come at great personal cost to individuals.
>
> (Layte *et al.* 2006, p. 123)

Insecurity on the part of lesbian and gay people in identifying themselves may be a result of the fact that at present in Ireland there is no legal recognition of same-sex relationships. This also leads to difficulties for those who have children. Within Irish law, as it is the woman who gives birth, it is she who can make decisions regarding the child's health care or schooling, irrespective of co-parenting by a partner. However, a 'Civil Partnership Bill' was published in June 2009 proposing to grant legal recognition to same-sex couples which is promised to be legalized by October 2010.

A brief review of lesbian women's experiences of health care

Over the last 25 years, research has been carried out on lesbian women's experience or perceived experiences of health care provision by health care providers (Marrazzo and Stine 2004). Lesbian women attend health care services less often than heterosexual women (Fields and Scout 2001). The reasons for non-access relate to ambivalence (White and Dull 1997), and/or lesbian women may not consider themselves to be exposed to the same risk factors for illness and infections as heterosexual women (Enszer 1996). Reagan (1981, p. 21) suggests the problems facing lesbian women are twofold: 'those that face women in general with dealing with the medical profession and those specific to being lesbian'. Lesbian women avoid health care services either from fear of discrimination or experience of judgements made by health care professionals on sexual identity and sexuality [sexual practice] (Marrazzo *et al.* 2005).

The issues uncovered in international health care research were reflected by Irish lesbian women in the first seminar held on lesbian health in 1999 (LEA and Western Health Board 1999). Eight concerns were identified which were reflected in the study by Gibbons *et al.* (2007) in the north-western region of Ireland. These issues included disclosure of sexual orientation, recognition of partnerships/next of kin, parenthood, mental health and sexual/gynaecological health (Gibbons *et al.* 2007).

Theoretical framework

I chose the hermeneutical or interpretative phenomenological perspective as the theoretical framework for my study as it 'fits' with my aim to explore the lived experience of lesbian women as consumers of health care. Whilst a total of 12 women were recruited for the study, in this chapter I present insights from five lesbian women's experiences of gynaecological health care.

The philosophy of Heidegger (1962), which was developed further by Sartre (1969), underpins this study. Heidegger's (1962) concern with being *in* the world (also refer to Chapters 3, 4 and 12), offers a theoretical frame-work whereby lesbian women can be seen as active participants in the world, creating understanding and meaning to their existence. Johnson (2000, p. 136) suggests that Heidegger views the human being (Dasein) as 'always involved in the practical world of experience'. As Heidegger (1962, p. 86) indicates 'Being-in-the-world is a basic state of Dasein'. Being-in-the-world of health care for lesbian women as service users is that of the outsider, rendering them vulnerable to the knowledgeable professionals (Sauliner 2002). Lesbian women's susceptibility in health care has been well documented in terms of judgements about sexual orientation (Marrazzo *et al.* 2005); age-related assumptions (Hinchliff *et al.* 2005) and use of hetero-sexual language (McDonald *et al.* 2003).

Sartre (1969) offers us a lens through which we can examine how lesbian women experience the self as service users. Sartre was interested in the question of subjectivity, suggesting that it was free, not constrained by religion or any other controlling factors, as an individual is not a means to an end, but an end itself. The individual must create her/himself. In particular I wanted to know how lesbian women remain lesbian within health care encounters. It is this capturing of life as it is lived, that frames the articulation of understanding and meanings that lesbian women derive from the situations they find themselves in.

Methodology

Following ethical approval from Dublin City University Ethics Committee, an advertisement to obtain a sample of lesbian women was placed in the *Gay Community News* (*GCN*) newspaper in March 2006. Data gathering took place between May 2006 and April 2007. During the initial enquiries from potential participants, we spoke about what my study was about and what I would like them to talk about. In this way they could think and reflect on their experiences in their own time and space, prior to the interview. The techniques chosen for the purpose of data collection were unstructured interviews. My status as an 'insider' researcher was made explicit by stating in the advertisement requesting study participants that I am a lesbian researcher. Initially in the data gathering process I wondered how much of myself I should give; however, it is the nature of research to give of the self (Letherby 2003). The interview process is a social interaction situation, and the more open I became about my own identity, the more relaxed and forthcoming the participants became. This was similar to other researchers in that lesbian or indeed gay participants are more informative to lesbian or gay researchers (Phellas 2000, McDermott 2004). As Kavanagh (2006) indicates 'it is in the co-disclosure of the shared world that issues of voice, reflexivity, identity, and understanding reveal themselves' (p. 252). A third of the analysed interviews (other participants declined to participate in this process) were sent back to the participants for verification.

The interview consisted of one question from which other questions or areas were explored as they arose. The question posed was: 'Could you please describe your experiences of health care?' Data analysis was guided by Heidegger's (1993) concept of dwelling, listening to the voices of lesbian women, moving forward in parts and taking refuge in other parts. Through writing and re-writing an interpretive text emerged.

Five women's experiences of seeking gynaecological services are presented in this chapter. These women were aged between 28 and 32 years. To disguise the identity of participants, pseudonyms of old Celtic Irish origin were used. They are known as Aibheann, Afric, Barrfind, Caireann and Folda.

Aibheann has a history of admissions for procedures emanating from gynaecological issues, which she indicated are part of her medical history, and the history of both her mother's and father's family. Afric and Caireann were seeking to start a family which led them to encountering gynaecological care. Barrfind and Folda were also seeking to begin their family and sought out assisted reproductive techniques in Ireland.

Limitations of the study

Hermeneutic phenomenology claims, meanings and understanding of everyday life 'are bound by context' (Estefan *et al.* 2004, p. 36). The findings of this study, conducted in Ireland in 2006 with a small number of participants, are not necessarily generalizable to other population groups. Van Manen (2002, p. 7) suggests hermeneutic phenomenology writing does 'not yield absolute truths, or objective observations', rather, 'at best gains an occasional glimpse of the meaning of human experience'. A phenomenological study is always 'one interpretation'. This study presents interpretations of the experiences of lesbian women, which were informed by the participants' narratives, as well as my own personal experiences of health care as a lesbian woman.

Findings

This section presents the themes that emerged from the interviews with lesbian women who sought gynaecological health care. The dominant theme is 'being different' in health care. The Irish women's health care strategy advocated woman-friendly health care, creating a service that 'should not further marginalise women who are already marginalised' (Government of Ireland 1997, p. 54). These findings consider whether this approach is being implemented, and are divided into six parts. The first deals with the experience of being different in a gynaecological health care setting; the second reviews the Sartrean concept of bad faith and its effect on lesbian patients; the third explores the issues of whether lesbian women can or cannot become parents; the fourth investigates the reality of becoming pregnant in Irish society; the fifth uncovers the emotional and financial choices of being different; and finally, the sixth unravels the experiences of isolation that emanates from being different.

Being different

Aibheann discussed her experience of obtaining gynaecological health care that had occurred in November 2005. Aibheann is 'out' (disclosure of sexual orientation) to her family, friends and co-workers. It is this open sense of self in relation to her sexuality that Aibheann brings with her when she is admitted to hospital. Aibheann had the expectation that the health care profession was aware of lesbian existence in Irish society. However, her expectations were shattered when the prejudice of her health care professional was disclosed:

> One of the registrars, when I was there, was talking to me and whatever and she was saying, when was the last time you had sex, and when was the last time you had intercourse, and when was the last time, and I'm not one to get embarrassed or anything like that, but then she started getting down to the nitty gritty, and I was just thinking this woman does not have a clue what it's like to be gay in this country, and have someone asking you questions like this. Then it came down to something very personal, and she said, and I was kind of out of it at this time probably as well, … I don't know what they gave me, but I think I was starting to float away and she said well have you ever had sex with a man and I went "why is it relevant", and she went "oh well I need to know". I went, "well no", and she said "oh well technically you're still a virgin" and I went "I'm sorry I'm what? Excuse me, can you just repeat what you just said" and she did. I was kind of there, whatever your perception of, I can't even remember what I said to her right now, but it wasn't very flattering, even though I kept my composure and didn't use any bad language, but I was not impressed. Not only did she bring this up on the first morning I was admitted, but everyday I was there she made reference to that, everyday I was there and this was last November [2005] and I couldn't believe it. I was there, who does this person think she is.
>
> (Aibheann)

Like other people, lesbian women are vulnerable when they are in hospital, and they expect that health care professionals have an understanding of their situation. Aibheann's story indicates some health care professionals are not only unaware of lesbianism, but are also openly prejudiced towards lesbian women. Aibheann's feeling of comfort as she was 'starting to float away' from the medication was brought back to the reality of the 'difference' in her situation. As Aibheann states above this was illustrated by reinforcing the heterosexual norm at every opportunity by Aibheann's doctor from the initial consultation, to every day of her hospital stay. Her health care provider pronounced with authority that lesbian sex is not real sex as it is not between a woman and a man. Aibheann's worth and value as a sexual human being is measured against the heterosexual norm. Consequently she felt devalued as a sexual human being as she states 'this woman does not have a clue what it's like to be gay in this country' (Aibheann). Her worth, value, and understandings of who she is in the world were undermined:

> It is only through being objectified that we can be given a value, assigned a worth, some 'thing' that can be assessed.
>
> (Howard 2002, p. 59)

Aibheann is not measured in accordance to her own community but to the general heterosexual community, the community of the assessor, which in this case is the health care provider. Within this measurement she becomes a virgin. Her sexual activities are relegated to non-existence:

> By far the most, you see that was the thing, what made me feel terrible was that morning in X [names urban hospital], it was almost like I felt ashamed to be gay, because this woman felt she could say that your sex life is completely irrelevant, because your partners have been female. I just thought what the hell is this woman on.
>
> (Aibheann)

Sartre (1969) suggests that 'shame of self; it is the recognition of the fact that I am indeed that object which the Other is looking at and judging' (p. 261). This gaze disrupts the sense of self, the taken-for-granted knowledge of knowing who I am. Aibheann did not allow herself to become the object of this judgement; rather she 'almost felt' but did not quite get there, as she questioned the ability of her health care provider to render her 'ashamed' of who she was.

Sartre (1969) suggests shame occurs once there is no freedom to be. Through questioning the validity of her health care provider to judge her, Aibheann reasserts her freedom to be. Although she is this being that the Other judges, a lesbian woman, she has embraced herself:

I am this self which another knows. And this self which I am – this I am in a world which the Other has made alien to me, for the Other's look embraces my being.

(Sartre 1969, p. 261)

The world as Aibheann understands it has disappeared from her and becomes a world that she does not recognize. Not only has the world become alien to her, she is simultaneously alienated from the world. However, she successfully prevents the alienation of the self. Aibheann had pointed out that she lived her life 'out' and 'open' to her family, work colleagues and friends. She was out of the closet and had no intention of going back there. This is why the power of the medical profession almost made her 'feel ashamed of being gay'.

Bad faith

Aibheann's sense of marginalization is further compounded when she discovers her health care provider was aware of lesbian existence within society:

> What made me more surprised was the next day then she was filling me in that her best friend and one of her colleagues in the hospital is in a female, same sex relationship, and that one of them is pregnant by a donor that they know. I was thinking OK in her private life she seems to be someway progressive and then at work she seems to be an absolute cow towards her patients, so I think that actually made me feel worse. I remember saying it to her the next day, I just said well I was a bit taken aback by what you mentioned yesterday and then for her to bring it up again and give her view again and then the next day to give her view, not only again to me, but to the doctor beside her, and it was almost like the cringe embarrassment factor with me there in the room again. I'm kind of going, it's almost like you're irrelevant, you are irrelevant if you're gay in this country and you go into a maternity hospital. She made me feel like Dr X, you're a waste of space, let me treat the heterosexual couple behind you.
>
> (Aibheann)

Aibheann attempts to understand and give meaning to her experience by questioning her health care provider's attitude towards lesbian women. She is surprised as she had attributed meaning to her health care provider's reactions as emanating through a lack of knowledge about lesbian life, and the possibility of never having encountered another lesbian woman.

Aibheann began to realize that there is a strict line between one's private life and one's professional life. Privately, some health care professionals may have friendships that include diversity in sexual orientation but publicly they reinforce the heterosexual norms of society. This could also be viewed as the recognition by the health care provider of the heteronormativity of the hospital setting (McDonald 2006). Equally, it represents the success of her medical training (Beagan 2000), the effectiveness of professional socialization (Mackintosh 2000), and the ability of the health care provider in reinforcing the norms, values and belief systems of their profession (Gibbons *et al.* 2007).

However from a Sartrean point of view the health care provider could be perceived as being in 'bad faith'. Sartre suggests that, through lying to both the self and others, the individual is avoiding the truth of the situation. The health care provider illustrates this by initially indicating to Aibheann that lesbian life was non-normative. She expresses the untruth of the situation, leading Aibheann to find some meaning for her provider's initial pronouncement. On the other hand, the health care provider could be said to be in 'bad faith' with her friend in that she does not view lesbian women's relationships as being equal to heterosexual relationships. When the health care provider reinforces her attitude towards lesbianism in front of another health care provider, she is the 'one who practises bad faith is hiding a displeasing truth or presenting as truth a pleasing untruth' (Sartre 1969, p. 49).

To be or not to be parents

The environment of the hospital differs to that of society, and this is where the reality of being a lesbian woman must be navigated as Aibheann's story illustrates. Aibheann became the Other in the eye of her health care provider. Two couples, Barrfind and Folda, and Caireann and Afric, recount their stories of trying to become parents. From within their stories it appeared that primary health care is one location where lesbian women can be themselves.

In Barrfind and Folda's case, Barrfind chose to be the person who would become pregnant in their quest to start a family. Folda begins their story:

> She [doctor] wasn't even surprised I don't think because the two of us went to the surgery together. … the two of us just walked into her room and she didn't seem fazed at all.
>
> (Folda)

Barrfind continues their story of the initial encounter with the primary health care team:

> She had a nurse there who did some research to find out if any of the clinics in Ireland would help us and she was very supportive. … I suppose we got this positive feeling from them.
>
> (Barrfind)

For both Barrfind and Folda sexual orientation was not an issue; they were able to be themselves and be together during their first consultation. They were offered the opportunity to be, that is not to feel different. The normality of their experience witnessed by the observation that 'she (health professional) wasn't even surprised' from the beginning of their quest. By being seen together the reality of the truth of their situation was acknowledged by the primary health care team.

In a similar way, Afric tells her story of seeking help for both herself and Caireann from her primary health care practitioner in their choice to become parents:

> I rang my GP [general practitioner] and I asked her if I could have an appointment to meet her for myself and my partner to chat to her about her ideas and what we could do about treatment in Ireland to have a baby basically. When I rang her at first I said about me and my partner so she assumed automatically that it was a guy and when I gave her Caireann, when I used the name obviously, so I said about myself and Caireann and she said absolutely perfect, come in and she was so supportive and delighted that I felt at ease contacting her. She was delighted that I was comfortable bringing Caireann and going myself obviously, coming to her and asking her advice, so that was really good. I was standing in a shopping centre when I made the phone call, I was on my own, I was down the country and she made me feel so good, like I was nearly skipping around the place, which was great.
>
> (Afric)

What Afric's story illustrates is that the initial contact with a health care provider can lead to positive feelings of the self. Afric, Barrfind and Folda's stories revealed that primary health care in Ireland has achieved a woman-friendly health care. It points to a health care service based on trust and mutual respect (Ward and Savulescu 2006), leading to the incorporation of the patient-as-person and doctor-as-person (Mead and Bower 2000). Within this service it was the health issues that were focused upon rather than the person presenting with a health care need. In this way, both couples experienced a patient-centred health service whereby the primary health care team were either educated practitioners (Albarran and Salmon 2000), or health care professionals, who could provide care regardless of their understanding of different modes of living (Naef 2006).

From a Heideggerian (1962) perspective, Afric, Barrfind and Folda experienced the authenticity of the self. Their quest to have a child opened to them the possibility to become authentic (Heidegger 1962). When Heidegger (1962) speaks of being authentic he suggests that it is a choice: I can choose my possibilities but I can also limit them. Folda, Barrfind and Afric chose their authenticity by seeing themselves as lesbian women seeking to become parents. As couples, both Barrfind and Folda, and Afric and Caireann, declared their authenticity by viewing Barrfind's or Afric's quest to become parents not only as belonging to them, but belonging to them as a couple. In this way they chose their possibility of becoming in whatever way their exploration to become parents took them. It became a part of who they were as a couple. As Sartre (1985, p. 44) indicates '[C]hoice always remains a choice in a situation' and that 'one makes a choice in relationship to others'.

Facing the reality of being different in Ireland

When these lesbian women initiated steps to obtain assisted reproduction health care, they discovered that they would have to go abroad as there were no clinics assisting lesbian couples in Ireland. O'Mathúna *et al.* (2005) suggest that health services should take steps to 'ensure that access to health care services is available without discrimination and on the basis of people's health care needs' (p. 133). It is clear that this has not been achieved for lesbian women who seek to become parents. In Ireland there is no legislation regulating the medical procedures of assisted reproduction. The lesbian couples in this study experienced that these procedures are available only to heterosexual couples.

Both couples recounted frustration and disappointment with the lack of medical procedures available to lesbian parents in Ireland:

> We decided to go down the clinic route which is not very easy in Ireland. I found out recently that actually there was no legislation as such.
>
> (Caireann)

> I suppose then in that process of trying to have a child and trying to get help in Ireland, there isn't any help, more or less. The frustration around that, why is it that we can't have this service in Ireland.
>
> (Barrfind)

These lesbian women thereby recognized that it was more or less the heterosexual couples who are considered first priority. This experience led Afric to acknowledge her difference:

> It's kind of like; I suppose for me, what I feel like jeez it should be available to us. Why can't it, like if there's a couple that can't have children, heterosexual couple.
>
> (Afric)

Afric views her situation as being similar to that of heterosexual couples who need reproductive assistance. The recognition that lesbian women are not afforded the same options exposes her difference. Folda on the other hand deems it as discriminatory in that heterosexuals obtain first priority in this particular area of health care. Becker (1963) suggested that homosexuals as a subculture in society 'have difficulty in any area of social activity in which assumption of normal sexual interests and propensities for marriage is made without question' (p. 35). This is the kernel of the problem for lesbian women seeking to become parents; the all-pervasive presumption of heterosexuality. It points to the power of the medical profession in this sector of health care to reinforce the sexual norms of society. Both couples experience their difference within a heterosexual society through their inability to receive assisted reproduction health care in Ireland. Sartre (1969, p. 260) suggests 'I see myself because somebody sees me'. However, in this case one could say, 'I see myself because nobody sees me'.

While neither of the lesbian women could be themselves in Irish health care, Barrfind indicates that the health care she received in another European country allowed her to be herself:

> That was fantastic because you arrived to a clinic where they treated other lesbian couples and you were like everyone else and you don't have to feel under pressure.
>
> (Barrfind)

Sartre (1969, p. 257) suggests that 'Being-seen-by-the-Other' is the truth of 'seeing-the-Other'. For the lesbian woman, the truth of being-seen-by-the-Other is that the Other knows who she is. Equally, to know the self is to know how the Other sees her. I no longer know the self as I see it, but rather I know it as the Other sees it, and I become the object for the Other and simultaneously become my own object. I am no longer the self as I view it and understand it, rather I have become the self as the Other sees it and understands it. Barrfind comprehends this and the clinic in Europe allows her and Folda to be comfortable with their 'self'.

The emotional and financial choices of being different

Folda, Barrfind, Caireann and Afric accessed European countries for reproductive care. Afric recounts how she found herself living a dual life during the period of seeking to become a parent. She did not want her private and public life overlapping. To maintain this she had to devise strategies which included 'lying to people' to obtain leave from work:

> So yeah to go to X [names city], well it's inconvenient, isn't it really? I mean you're trying to, and how I feel about the whole thing, it's inconvenient, you've to lie to people. People that I work with I have to lie to them to try and organise time off and being the person that's not carrying the baby, it's very difficult if you're trying to keep your private life private because you're trying to say you've a doctor's appointment, but how can your doctor's appointment run for 2 days, so it's very difficult. Also the stress levels, it's extremely stressful.
>
> (Afric)

Afric found she could not be truthful about her situation in her work-place. The truth of her situation appears to be that she is a lesbian woman who does not fit into the life realities that surround her. As a result, Afric became socially isolated from her peers. Afric could have chosen not to lie and tell her colleagues but she made a choice not to. Sartre (1985, p. 44) indicates '[C]hoice always remains a choice in a situation'. She made the choice in the situation she was confronted with. As described earlier, Sartre (1985 p. 44) believed that 'one makes a choice in relationship to others'. In this story, Afric made a choice in relation to Others but also in relation to herself. So could Afric choose to say nothing? Sartre (1985, p. 39) provides us with a way out of this conundrum of whether we are making a choice to tell the truth or lie: '[C]hoice is possible, but what is not possible is not to choose. I can always choose, but I ought to know that if I do not choose, I am still choosing'. Therefore, Afric is still making a choice: in Sartrean terms I can choose one way or another. In other words, Afric either chooses to tell the truth or lie. It is a conscious decision made by her.

Barrfind is aware of the burden of the expense of receiving treatment outside of Ireland:

> We have to spend a heap of money and travel a great distance to get a service that's available to other people.
>
> (Barrfind)

Barrfind finds meaning in this situation through recognizing her differ-ence to Others. She perceives that heterosexual couples do not incur the expenditure she and Folda had to, due to the privileges associated with het-erosexuality. Caireann on the other hand becomes vulnerable as she finds there is not a set price – rather it is a shifting reality:

> The fact that we knew from the beginning that we had a list of prices and we knew exactly what we were getting into, but then there were hidden costs. When I was basically in the room with the nurse that was going to do the insemination, I was told 'oh by the way I heard today that we're going to have to charge you another Y just to have a look at the scans'. What do you say, I mean once you've travelled over to X [names the city] and the two of us were doing that all the time together so it was double price basically, you multiply everything by two and you get there and then you're told in that room, when you go to lie down and get the insemination done, that basically you're going to have to spend another Y. What can you say, of course yes fine, just go ahead and do it.
>
> (Caireann)

In this account Caireann and Afric knew what their outlay would be, and had calculated for that. However, it is the changing circumstances that render

Caireann feeling unhappy, vulnerable and ill-at-ease. She was informed at a time when saying 'no' was not an option as she was about to be inseminated. Shildrick (2002) points out that 'Vulnerability, [is] an existential state that may belong to any one of us, but which is characterised nonetheless as a negative attribute, a failure to self-protection, that opens the self to the potential of harm' (p. 1). For both these couples their vulnerability lay in their wish to become parents and they found themselves open to services that could fix their prices or have fluidity in their pricing arrangements. From Caireann's story it would appear that if you want a child you will pay whatever the price is today.

Isolation and being different

Afric expressed her feelings of isolation about her difference when she said:

> So everything is over in 4 or 5 minutes and you're up and gone, walking down the street. Although there are two of you, you feel alone. Has anyone realised what you have been through? There's all those things run through your head as you sit on a train in X or wherever watching around you. It's a bit surreal, the whole experience.
>
> (Afric)

Afric experiences isolation and aloneness in her situation as a direct result of her sexuality. Even though she is surrounded by people out in the street and in the train station she is alone in the world with her thoughts. She feels different to them. Heidegger (1962) suggests that even if there are Others around us present-to-hand, 'Dasein can still be alone' (p. 157). Dasein refers to the human being in the world who is 'always involved in the practical world of experience" (Johnson 2000, p. 136). Heidegger (1962) indicates that even if we are 'among them' we encounter them 'in a mode in which they are indifferent and alien' (p. 157).

Indifference, for Heidegger, relates the way in which we pass one another by. In public places Afric discovers that the world is indifferent to her. However, it could be argued that she too is indifferent to them as she is equally passing them by. While Afric is a Being-in-the-world, so too are those around her. However, Heidegger (1962) suggests that Being-alone is still Being-with in the world. We cannot feel Being-alone outside the Being-with-Others. In other words, Afric experiences her aloneness as Being-with-Others; she does not live through aloneness when she is on her own because she has the support of those who know her completely, such as her friends and family in Ireland. Equally, from a Heideggerian point of view, Afric's aloneness is a closing off of her self to Others. She denies herself the possibility of being open to the Other and the relationship of Being-with-Being. She does this by not sharing her feelings and thoughts with Caireann, as even though 'there are two of you, you feel alone'.

Summary of the findings

While Aibheann experienced a 'non-friendly' women's health care service, there is an area according to the experience of Afric, Barrfind, Caireann and Folda that seems to have achieved a woman-friendly health care, namely primary health care. Within the primary health care service, the truth of the lived experience can come to the fore. It points to a service that is based on trust and mutual respect (Ward and Savulescu 2006), leading to the incorporation of the patient-as-person (Mead and Bower 2000). Within this service it was the health care needs that were focused upon rather than the person presenting. This led to lesbian women experiencing the authenticity of the self with all the possibilities of becoming (Heidegger 1962).

Lesbian women report experiences of 'being different' in health care encounters. However, they experience their difference both as patients from other patients, and from those who are providers of health care, whether they are doctors or nurses in a health care setting. While their differences are exposed for both themselves as lesbian women and Others to see, Heidegger (1962) suggests there is always a possibility to become, that is, I am not finite, I am constantly becoming through a reflective process of my situation. Therefore, lesbian women find meaning and understanding in both their situation as well as in who they are in their day-to-day interactions within society, which they bring into health care. Dasein, that is, the human being in the world, exists within society (Heidegger 1962) and through interconnectedness, the lesbian woman becomes whoever she is by making a choice (Sartre 1985) whether to come out or not. While a lesbian woman knows her difference, she decides whether to expose it to Others. However, there are times where she feels that she does not have a choice through constraints of her personal situation.

Implications

The Health Service Executive (HSE) has the responsibility 'to improve, promote and protect the health and welfare of the public' (www.hse.ie). It is therefore the responsibility of the HSE to promote and provide adequate health care provision for lesbian women. It is the policy of the Irish government that all health services were directed to develop an action plan to 'ensure that health professionals are informed about lesbian health issues', and that all health care staff were to 'respect the sexual orientation of lesbian women (Government of Ireland 1997, p. 64). This policy lays down the type of action that needs to be undertaken to create woman-friendly health care, reviewing staff attitudes, and developing training programmes for sensitivity. This would suggest that information, *per se*, will not enable health care professionals to change attitudes and training programmes also need to be implemented. While the findings of this study would suggest that the HSE needs to review its staff training, the primary health care exhibited an ability to recognize lesbian relationships. This would suggest that other health care services can be created that incorporate the patient-as-person, thus recognizing the patient as being-in-the-world, bringing with her all facets that make up personhood into health care.

Conclusion

This chapter illustrates how lesbian women understand and give meaning to the situations in which they find themselves in a health setting context. Their stories exemplify attempts to reconcile the self with a culture of health care based upon heterosexuality. This reflects initial studies (Cochran and Mays 1988; Reagan 1981) and later studies (Hinchliff *et al.* 2005, Gibbons *et al.* 2007) which report that diversity in women's sexuality is not recognized in health care settings.

Heidegger (1962) and Sartre (1969) provide a theoretical framework from which the meanings and understanding of lesbian women in the world of health care can be interpreted. Findings generated through this lens suggest that the aspiration of creating a woman-friendly health care service for lesbian women has not yet been fully achieved in Ireland.

Acknowledgement

This study was part-funded by the Irish Research Council for Humanities and Social Science Postgraduate Scholarship 2006–2007.

References

Albarran J. W. and Salmon D. (2000) Lesbian, gay and bisexual experiences within critical care nursing, 1988–1998: A survey of the literature. *International Journal of Nursing Studies* 37, 445–455.

Beagan B. L. (2000) Neutralizing differences: producing neutral doctors for (almost) neutral patients. *Social Science and Medicine* 51, 1253–1265.

Becker, Howard S. (1963) *Outsiders: Studies in the Sociology of Deviance.* The Free Press: New York.

Cochran S. D. and Mays V. M. (1988) Disclosure of sexual preference to physicians by black lesbian and bisexual women. *The Western Journal of Medicine* 149 (5), 616–619.

Enszer J. R. (1996) *Health Care Needs of Lesbians: Issues and Access: A Report on the Lesbian and Bisexual Women's Health Survey.* Affirmations Lesbian/gay Community Center: USA.

Estefan A., McAllister M. and Rowe J. (2004) Difference, dialogue, dialectics; A study of caring and self-harm. In *Many Voices: Towards Caring Culture in Healthcare and Healing: Interpretive Studies in Healthcare and in Human Sciences* (eds Kavanagh K. H. and Knowlden V.), 21–61. The University of Wisconsin Press: Madison.

Fields C. B. and Scout M. A. (2001) Addressing the needs of lesbian patients. *Journal of Sex Education and Therapy* 26 (3), 182–188.

94   *Mel Duffy*

Gibbons M., Manandhar M., Gleeson C. and Mullan J. (2007) *Recognising LGB Sexual Identities in Health Services: The Experiences of Lesbian, Gay and Bisexual People with Health Services in North West Ireland.* The Equality Authority and the Health Service Executive. Brunswick Press: Dublin.

Government of Ireland (1997) *A Plan for Women's Health: 1997–99.* Stationary Office: Dublin.

Health Service Executive. Online at http://www.hse.ie. Last accessed 11 August 2010.

Heidegger M. (1962) *Being and Time* (translated by John Macquarrie and Edward Robinson) Harper and Row Publishers: New York.

Heidegger M. (1993) Building Dwelling Thinking. In *Martin Heidegger: Basic Writings* (ed. Krell D.), 343–363. Harper: San Francisco.

Hinchliff S., Gott M. and Galena E. (2005) 'I daresay I might find it embarrassing': General Practitioners' perspectives on discussing sexual health issues with lesbian and gay patients. *Health and Social Care in the Community*, 13 (4), 345–353.

Howard P. (2002) 'The Look' in teacher's performance evaluation. In *Writing in the Dark: Phenomenological Studies in Interpretive Inquiry* (ed. van Manen M.). The Althouse Press: Canada.

Hug C. (1999) *The Politics of Sexual Morality in Ireland.* Macmillan Press: London.

Johnson M. E. (2000) Heidegger and Meaning: Implications for Phenomenological Research. *Nursing Philosophy* 1, 134–146.

Kavanagh K. H. (2006) Beyond the Individual: Healthcare Ethics in Diverse Societies. In *Listening to the Whispers: Re-thinking Ethics in Healthcare* (eds Sorrell Dinkins C. and Sorrell J. M.), 248–304. Madison: The University of Wisconsin Press.

Kenny M. (1997) *Goodbye to Catholic Ireland: A Social, Personal and Cultural History from the Fall of Parnell to the Realm of Mary Robinson.* Sinclair-Stevenson: London, Auckland, Melbourne, Singapore and Toronto.

Layte R., McGee H., Quail A., Rundle K., Cousins G., Donnelly C., Mulcahy F. and Conroy R. (2006) *The Irish Study of Sexual Health and Relationships.* Department of Health and Children and Crisis Pregnancy Agency: Dublin.

LEA and Western Health Board (1999) *Towards a More Inclusive Health Service: Report on a Seminar on Lesbian and Bisexual Health Services.* LEA and Western Health Board: Galway.

Lehmann J. B., Lehmann C. U. and Kelly P. J. (1998) Development and health care needs of lesbians. *Journal of Women's Health*, 7 (3), 379–387.

Lemon G. and Patton W. (1997) Lavender Blue: Issues in Lesbian Identity Development with a Focus on an Australian Lesbian Community. *Women's Studies International Forum*, 20 (1), 113–127.

Letherby G. (2003) *Feminist Research in Theory and Practice.* Buckingham: Open University Press.

Mackintosh C. (2000) Is there a place for 'care' within nursing? *International Journal of Nursing Studies* 37 (4), 321–327.

Marrazzo J. M. and Stine K. (2004) Reproductive health history of lesbians: Implications for care. *American Journal of Obstetrics and Gynecology*, 190, 1298–1304.

Marrazzo J. M., Coffey P. and Bingham A. (2005) Sexual practices, risk perception and knowledge of sexually transmitted disease risk among lesbian and bisexual women. *Perspectives on Sexual and Reproductive Health*, 37 (1), 6–12.

McDermott E. (2004) Telling Lesbian Stories: Interviewing and the Class Dynamics of 'Talk'. *Women's Studies International Forum* 27, 177–187.

McDonald C. (2006) Lesbian disclosure: Disrupting the taken for granted. *Canadian Journal of Nursing Research* 38 (1), 42–57.

McDonald C., McIntyre M. and Anderson B. (2003) The view from somewhere: locating lesbian experience in women's health. *Health Care for Women International*, 24, 697–711.

Mead N. and Bower P. (2000) Patient-centredness: A conceptual framework and review of the empirical literature. S*ocial Science and Medicine* 51, 1087–1110.

Naef R. (2006) Bearing witness: A moral way of engaging in the nurse-person relationship. *Nursing Philosophy* 7, 146–156.

Norman J., Galvin M. and McNamara G. (2006) *Straight Talk: Researching Gay and Lesbian Issues in the School Curriculum.* Centre for Education Evaluation: Dublin.

O'Mathúna D. P., Scott P. A., McAuley A., Walsh-Daneshmandi A. and Daly B. (2005) *Health Care Rights and Responsibilities: A Review of the European Charter of Patients Rights.* Irish Patients' Association: Dublin.

Phellas C. N. (2000) Cultural and Sexual Identities in In-Depth Interviewing. In *Research and Inequalities* (eds Truman C., Mertens D. M. and Humphries B.), 52–64. University College London Press: Dublin.

Reagan P. (1981) The interaction of health professionals and their lesbian clients. *Patient Counselling and Health Education* 3, 21–25.

Sartre. J.-P. (1969) *Being and Nothingness: An Essay on Phenomenological Ontology* (translated by Barnes H) Routledge: London.

Sartre, J.-P. (1985) *Existentialism and Human Emotions.* New York: Citadel Press, Kensington Publishing Corp.

Sauliner C. F. (2002) Deciding who to see: lesbians discuss their preferences in health and mental health care providers. *Social Work* 47, 355–365.

Shildrick M. (2002) *Embodying the Monster: Encounters with the Vunerable Self.* Sage Publications: London.

Taylor B. (1999) 'Coming out' as a life transition: homosexual identity formation and its implications for health care practice. *Journal of Advanced Nursing* 30 (2), 520–525.

van Manen M. (2002) *Writing in the Dark: Phenomenological Studies in Interpretive Inquiry.* The Althouse Press: Ontario.

Ward M. and Savulescu J. (2006) Patients who challenge. *Best Practice and Research Clinical Anaesthesiology* 20 (4), 545–563.

White J. C. and Dull V. T. (1997) Health risk factors and health-seeking behaviour in lesbians. *Journal of Women's Health* 6 (1), 103–112.

6   Women's lived experiences of severe early onset preeclampsia
A hermeneutic analysis

Joyce Cowan, Elizabeth Smythe and Marion Hunter

Introduction

In this chapter I describe a recent hermeneutic phenomenological study that I conducted to answer the question 'What are women's experiences of preeclampsia before 34 weeks of gestation?' Eight women who had experienced severe preeclampsia were interviewed during a 12-month period between 2003 and 2004, and their narratives analysed to uncover the meaning of the lived experience of preeclampsia from onset of symptoms to postpartum recovery. The analysis was informed by the writings of Martin Heidegger (1962/1927) and van Manen (1990). This chapter focuses on the 'showing of preeclampsia' as the disease progresses, and reveals the often unpredictable and complex manner in which symptoms occur. The findings of the study indicate that there are many atypical presentations and that sometimes the early 'showing' goes unrecognized. By considering each woman's individual risk profile, weighing up the likelihood of preeclampsia, and responding appropriately to the 'showing', it is more likely that timely diagnosis will be made and the risks for mother and baby reduced.

Justification for the study

At the commencement of this research there were no studies identified in the literature that explored the experiences of women who suffer preeclampsia, although research about the disease itself is well represented in medical and midwifery literature. In my role as director of the charity New Zealand Action on Preeclampsia (NZAPEC) many women who have experienced the disease have approached me. I have become aware of a need for these women to have a voice. Their case studies appear in the literature and their physiological responses to disease become part of the growing body of scientific research but their lived experience is seldom spoken or heard, apart from the stories they tell for the NZAPEC newsletters and consumer literature. I have heard many such stories over the years of my involvement with NZAPEC and was keen to take the opportunity to listen in depth, ask more questions and engage in a phenomenological analysis.

Historical context

Until the late nineteenth century practitioners had little understanding of preeclampsia and the associated mortality was considerable, even with the attendance of experienced obstetricians. For Evelina, one of the daughters of the renowned nineteenth century London banker, Lionel Rothschild, preeclampsia could neither be anticipated nor treated as this tragic account by Weintraub (2003) recounts:

> In the first stages of labour on Tuesday, December 4, 1866, Evelina was seized with convulsions. Arthur Farre, also obstetrician to the Princess of Wales, summoned two additional physicians, who could only assist in delivering a stillborn son. Minutes later Evelina was dead.
>
> (p. 207)

Family correspondence records that Evelina had apparently been well until the day before when her mother spent time with her, as she was a little uncomfortable. Almost 150 years later preeclampsia remains a complex, baffling and unpredictable syndrome. The condition affects the lives of approximately one in every 20 pregnant women. Most cases are mild but some are serious enough to threaten the life of mother and baby. Medical research has yet to identify a cause, and the search for a cure continues. Childbirth remains the only method of resolving this serious complication of pregnancy and may need to be effected before the fetus has become mature enough to avoid the risks associated with preterm birth.

The disease of preeclampsia

The aetiology of preeclampsia remains poorly understood, although there are several theories including genetic predisposition, immunological factors and defective trophoblast invasion resulting in reduced placental perfusion (Redman and Sargent 2005). Defective placentation is involved with a maternal response involving multiple physiological disturbances (Baker and Kingdom 2004). The underlying pathology is complex and clinical presentation varies extremely widely.

In many cases preeclampsia causes no symptoms until the mother or baby is very ill. Most cases are mild and occur close to full term with minimal maternal and perinatal risk, but in severe preeclampsia women are at risk of multi-organ failure and death (Duley *et al.* 2006), and their babies are at risk of intrauterine growth restriction, intrauterine death and complications of prematurity. In most cases the interests of mother and baby coincide when delivery is indicated but tragically it is sometimes necessary to deliver a woman for her own safety at the expense of a baby who is too premature to survive (Serenius *et al.* 2004).

Ideally, women would be diagnosed with the disease at a point when their birth can be induced in time to prevent serious complications, but the reality is that the disease can fulminate with little warning. Preeclampsia may also be diagnosed for the first time after childbirth (Matthys *et al.* 2004). The variability of preeclampsia makes diagnosis challenging and women are often shocked and ill-prepared for diagnosis.

There is currently no effective screening test to ensure that all women are diagnosed with preeclampsia early enough to prevent serious complications, although current international research (the SCOPE study) is underway to identify molecular and clinical markers that differentiate, early in pregnancy, women at high risk for the development of preeclampsia. Other research is in progress to develop a predictive test (Sunderji *et al.* 2010).

In the meantime, practitioners must remain vigilant for signs of the disease, which presents with a wide diversity of signs and symptoms. This study seeks to reveal some of the complexity of vigilance as revealed through the women's accounts.

Research design and methodology

My research question was 'What is woman's experience of severe early onset preeclampsia?'

Prejudices and pre-understandings

I was mindful of my own prejudices and possible biases (Gadamer 1982/1960) that came with me in my analysis. Some years earlier I had been involved in the care of a woman who very nearly died through preeclampsia. That was a defining experience in my life, leading me to initiate a New Zealand branch of the group founded by Professor Christopher Redman and medical journalist Isobel Walker, UKAPEC (Action on Preeclampsia). I thus have a passion to do whatever I can to keep women and their babies who experience preeclampsia safe, and to ensure practitioners are as knowledgeable as possible as to how to provide safe care. Wendy Roberts, (Cowan 1997) wrote of her feelings on returning home after six weeks in hospital during which time she suffered multiple organ failure and disseminated intravascular coagulation:

> Day by day I gained more strength to enable me to finally come home... the home we had made for Finn to grow up in. My initial reaction was to cry. I realized that I may never have set foot in this house again, never seen grass so green and sky so blue and my cat – so loving and full of personality and my friend, our baby – my lifelong dream. And, of course and most importantly, my cherished husband, who was at my side every day and night for the entire time I was in hospital and every day since this ordeal – sometimes I think I could not have got through

this without him. He was a tower of strength. But when it all boils down to it, we are all fragile creatures, we need to be loved and life is for living and loving.

(Cowan 1997)

Philosophical approach

Phenomenological research as an interpretive methodology concerned with understanding phenomena that are part of human experience seemed to 'fit' my study. In particular, my work was informed by Heidegger (1962/1927) who was concerned with the phenomenology of human being, or Dasein (also discussed in Chapters 3, 8 and 12). 'Phenomenological description, as a method, lies in interpretation' (p. 61). A Heideggerian notion which leaped out and caught my attention as being perfectly suited to the study of women's experience of preeclampsia was Heidegger's (1962/1927) notion of phenomenon as 'What lies in the light of day or can be brought to the light' (p. 51). Preeclampsia may be present as a disease affecting a pregnant woman or her unborn baby for some time before diagnosis. The challenge lies in seeing and recognizing what must eventually be brought to light. The disease may show itself or may appear as a semblance of 'something, which it is not' (p. 52). The difficulties experienced with timely diagnosis are illustrated in the participants' stories. The phenomenon of preeclampsia may exist but may not be recognized when it 'shows itself as itself' or as 'a semblance of itself' thus presenting a challenge to caregivers.

Participants

Eight women were recruited for this study by purposive and snowballing methods. Inclusion criteria for this study were that women had experienced severe preeclampsia at less than 34 weeks of pregnancy and that they were fluent in English. All women were European and with two exceptions had experienced severe early onset preeclampsia in their first pregnancies. Gestation at diagnosis of preeclampsia ranged from 24 weeks to 37 weeks; although the woman diagnosed at 37 weeks had experienced symptoms of preeclampsia for several weeks before diagnosis. All babies were delivered by emergency caesarean section. One baby died from complications of extreme prematurity and one baby has slight developmental delay. Interviews were conducted in the women's own homes with the exception of one which was conducted by telephone. A conversational approach was used in which women were simply encouraged to tell their story.

Ethical issues

Ethical approval was obtained from the Auckland Ethics committee. Throughout my study I was aware of the need to protect the rights of participants, particularly as there was a potential for distressing memories to be triggered during interviews. My ethics application included a personal commitment to provide for the cost of counselling for participants should the need become apparent during the research process.

Staying mindful of the need to remain close to my research question, I commenced each interview with an open-ended question such as 'Please tell me about your experience with preeclampsia starting from when you were first aware that you were unwell'. From there participants would talk quite freely. I occasionally asked for clarification with a question such as 'Could you please explain what that felt like to you?' It was rarely necessary to bring the woman back to the topic, as invariably the research question was the focus of her recalled story. Although participants experienced some distress while talking about their experiences, the need for counselling did not arise. In all cases the women were very willing to talk about their experiences and when given the opportunity to discontinue the interview if painful memories were triggered, all opted to continue after a short break as they wanted to share what had happened to them. The interviews were unstructured and lasted from one to two hours. I requested a second interview with one woman as she had a lot of painful experiences to share and I felt that lengthening the initial session would have been too hard for her. She was very positive about being available for a second interview some weeks later.

Analysis

One of the purposes of the interview in hermeneutic human science according to van Manen (1990) is '…exploring and gathering experiential narrative material that may serve as a resource for developing a richer and deeper understanding of a human phenomenon' (p. 66) (detailed insights into this approach are provided by Dowling in Chapter 4). From the first interview I was aware that the women were sharing with me insights that I would have not had without being involved in this study and I felt very grateful for the commitment that they showed to my study by being so willing to share their experiences in an open and in-depth manner. Kleiman (2004) discusses a relationship of dialogical openness between researcher and participant, with the researcher ready to allow the participant to speak and ready to listen. 'It is in fact this proffered readiness to listen that inspires participants to relate what presents itself to their consciousness in the immediate situation.' (p. 5). As interviews surprised me with new insights I made entries into a reflective journal.

Stories were crafted from the transcripts (Caelli 2001) to draw forth the meaning. These were returned to the participants to ensure the meaning was unchanged, and to allow them to delete or change anything. Using van Manen's (1990) thematic analysis I aimed to uncover the meaning within the stories the women told of their experiences. This involved writing interpretations of each story as a process of drawing forth understanding. As the writing progressed, so the themes began to emerge. Re-writing brought a sharper clarity. Ultimately the project of phenomenological reflection and explication is to effect a more direct contact with the experience as lived (van Manen 1990, p. 78). Reflection led me to a deeper understanding of my research question. However, interpretation was not necessarily the final step in the research process as I found that insights occurred at each stage from data collection to the final stages of analysis. I am also aware that understanding can never be complete. Gadamer (1982/1960) said, 'Discovery of true meaning is never finished, it is an infinite process' (p. 265).

Limitations

Although it can be considered that a limitation of a phenomenological study is that it may not provide findings that are generalizable to other settings (Crotty 1998), the experiences of the eight women who were interviewed have provided deep insights into what it is like to have a pregnancy complicated by severe preeclampsia.

Findings: the showing of preeclampsia

The findings of this study indicate that there are many atypical presentations of preeclampsia and that sometimes early 'showing' goes unrecognized. The woman may in fact feel better as the disease progresses. Late diagnosis leaves the woman and her family shocked and may compromise fetal and maternal safety. Having preeclampsia changes the reality of pregnancy and early parenting for a woman. Emotional consequences are significant and include an increased risk of post-traumatic stress disorder.

Diagnosis of preeclampsia at a time that is optimal in terms of maternal and fetal wellbeing is a challenge for the midwife or doctor. The disease may 'show' itself in many ways, some obvious, some atypical and confusing. Symptoms may hint that something is wrong. They may come and go. They may be confusing. Or they may suddenly announce the disease with frightening urgency. Heidegger (1962/1927) defines 'appearances or symptoms of an illness' as occurrences in the body that show themselves and in the self-showing 'indicate' something that does *not* show itself. (p. 25). The possibility of this self-showing looking like something else as a 'semblance' of another disease process may be problematic (Heidegger 1962/1927). This inconsistent and varied presentation of the disease is a great challenge for pregnant women and their caregivers. It was the realization that something was different, something was wrong, from which the 'showing' of preeclampsia was explored.

The disease hints

Evelyn was the one participant whose 'hinting' of preeclampsia was typical in that her blood pressure started to increase several weeks before she was diagnosed with the disease. She recalled the first time she became aware of the possibility of preeclampsia:

> It was around about my 28th week and my midwife had been checking my blood pressure regularly. She picked up that my blood pressure had risen slightly and just sort of made mention of it and referred me to an obstetrician. He just went over what preeclampsia is, and didn't necessarily say that was what it was going to be. So it was just kept an eye on basically, and then, a month later I was referred back to him, around about 31 weeks, and my blood pressure had gone up further; I also had 1+ of protein in my urine...
>
> (Evelyn)

This example illustrates a type of 'self showing' indicating that preeclampsia may be developing. The first symptom appeared before the woman was really unwell and there was then an indication to watch vigilantly for further signs and symptoms. This type of 'showing' makes diagnosis and management of preeclampsia relatively straightforward for the maternity caregiver. Progress is reasonably predictable and there is time to watch and wait with the awareness that intervention will be likely at some stage in the future.

The disease confuses

Other examples suggest that preeclampsia may be considerably less predictable and may initially confuse both women and caregivers, sometimes leading to potentially dangerous delays in diagnosis. Kate felt that something was wrong for several weeks before she was diagnosed with severe preeclampsia at 29 weeks:

> At about 20 weeks I started getting some oedema. By about 25 weeks my mother was getting quite concerned about how much oedema I had and how I was feeling. By about 26, 27 weeks I could leave really deep thumbprints of oedema all the way up to mid calf. I didn't feel great, I was really tired, and I just felt really gungy. It's hard to describe, but I guess kind of fluey feeling – I don't know if that's how I would describe it but I generally didn't feel well. With the oedema I was finding mobility difficult as well. I had so much oedema. Mum was worried about that as well. My face had suddenly ballooned since the previous time she saw me. That really triggered her concern and John's as well. I think I looked really sick. I was very tired and run down for about 4 weeks before Lilly was delivered.
>
> (Kate)

Kate experienced the general malaise common to women who are becoming sick with severe preeclampsia. Her oedema was severe, especially so early in pregnancy and she was finding it hard to walk and function generally. Family members are more likely than the midwife to be aware of 'the showing' of preeclampsia in the middle trimester because antenatal visits are often monthly. Perhaps they will notice facial oedema that the woman may not have recognized or encourage her to contact her midwife with any concerns.

This highlights the need to educate women early in pregnancy about the symptoms that indicate the need for urgent assessment. Women with severe preeclampsia frequently describe a feeling of 'unwellness' which may be attributed to a viral infection or physiological changes in pregnancy. Such a showing is a 'semblance'. It may seem that a woman 'just feeling unwell' has a condition such as the 'flu'. Consequently the preeclampsia remains hidden and unrecognized until another time.

Lynda, who had experienced preeclampsia in two previous pregnancies, was 24 weeks pregnant when she started to feel unwell with flu-like symptoms:

> It all went well until about 24 weeks, then I started getting backaches, quite high between my shoulder blades. I was just feeling like crap, having a bad day for a day, and then it would go away for 2 or 3 days and then come back. I had headaches, no energy whatsoever, just like I had been knocked about really badly. The pain came on at night and I felt my bed was really, really uncomfortable. I could not lie on anything and be comfortable. It was like something suddenly changed. In hindsight I remember I felt quite bad with my first baby Scott but I didn't connect it, because I had no problems with blood pressure or protein or anything. With him I remember feeling really in pain, like there was no relief. I got in and out of the bath twice trying to relieve the pain. It was just like a bad flu you know.
>
> (Lynda)

When Lynda started to experience symptoms of preeclampsia she did not connect her pain with her symptoms, which heralded the onset of the disease in a previous pregnancy. Perhaps she did not want to acknowledge to herself that her pregnancy was becoming complicated. Perhaps the pain was so strong and she felt so unwell that rational thought was precluded. She may also have discounted the possibility of preeclampsia occurring at such an early gestation. After several episodes of intense pain Lynda rang her midwife for advice:

> I got these wicked backaches, but I didn't know what it was. I rang my midwife, and she said it was just a virus, so I went back to bed, and the next day I felt OK. Four days later it came back again. It was only in

hindsight that I realized that it was a similar thing to with Scott but it wasn't obvious because I had no problems with blood pressure or pro-tein or anything. I think the third time it happened I went to the doctor crying, thinking it must be a kidney infection after I looked through the books that I had – which wasn't much – but I thought it's got to be something, you can't just tell me it's a virus, you know – recurring at intervals like that. The doctor took my blood pressure and told me it was high.

(Lynda)

When Lynda experienced the pain for a second time she didn't seek advice from her midwife. How are midwives to 'know' when something is wrong when the woman does not report back with continuing symptoms? Lynda had been told four days previously that her symptoms were probably due to a virus and therefore she might have been reluctant to re-contact her mid-wife. How can midwives ensure that their clients feel free to contact them if concerned, without risk of feeling that they are over-reacting?

The disease hides

It is interesting to consider what might be happening to a woman and her baby in the times when the symptoms disappear, even when they have been severe. The disease itself does not disappear in those times but appears to hide in the absence of symptoms, potentially confusing both the woman and her caregivers.

By the third time the pain returned Lynda knew that something was wrong, she thought, 'It's got to be something' and assessed herself as pos-sibly having a urinary infection after consulting her books. Linda elected to see her GP who found that her blood pressure was high:

He was mildly concerned about it, did the urine test and gave me anti-biotics for a possible kidney infection. He asked me to see my midwife in three more days for another blood pressure check.

(Lynda)

It appears that the GP was not sufficiently concerned about the increase in blood pressure to order any blood tests that may have led to a diagnosis of preeclampsia. However, he did ask Lynda to see her midwife for a further blood pressure check in three days time. There is a risk in not being in step with the potential rapid progress of preeclampsia.

The disease suddenly announces itself

Paradoxically, the disease may be progressing rapidly even though the woman is less symptomatic or even feeling well:

> I went to see the midwife on the way to work. It was strange, I was feeling better by then but my blood pressure was 180/100 or something like that! The midwife took it, she sat down, took it on my other arm and then she took her own blood pressure with the same machine! By this time I thought – 'Uh-oh – I'm in trouble now'.
>
> (Lynda)

Perhaps the midwife did not believe the blood pressure reading and hence tested it again and then took her own blood pressure with the same machine. Perhaps she did not want to have to tell Lynda that her pregnancy was probably now seriously complicated, with the consequent fear and distress the woman may experience. As 'guardians of normal birth' midwives may feel disappointment when a pregnancy becomes abnormal and may tend to want to 'normalize the abnormal' or protect the woman from the knowledge that things are not going well, but primarily aim to ensure that a suspected complication and referral is based on accurate information. Lynda was actually feeling better at this stage and might have looked to the midwife for confirmation that all was well. This is how it can appear to 'hide' when symptoms disappear and 'confuse' the woman and possibly her caregivers. However, the preeclampsia was by now announcing itself clearly and prompt action was necessary. It appears that Lynda's 'Uh-oh' signifies that she certainly recognized that she now had the condition yet again.

The disease slowly reveals itself

Sarah had a greatly increased risk of developing preeclampsia in her first pregnancy as she was expecting twins, had a family history of preeclampsia, an IVF pregnancy and gestational diabetes. At 32 weeks she was admitted for investigation of abdominal pain and malaise and discharged when the results of investigations were normal:

> Everything was perfectly normal with my pregnancy until about 32 weeks. I then developed some right upper abdominal pain which was so bad at one stage I rang the on-call obstetrician and went into the assessment unit. The pain was quite sharp, I had also had some vomiting and diarrhoea, felt generally unwell and hot. They did tests for Listeria and some liver function blood tests but they came back normal. They suggested the pain could have been caused by one of the babies kicking me or perhaps I could have had a gallstone and suggested that I have my liver scanned during the next ultrasound examination.
>
> Over the next 2 weeks the pain got worse and definitely felt like liver pain. It was right under my ribs, almost like my ribs were being squashed in, quite uncomfortable especially at night. I didn't have any swelling except a little in my fingers, but did have a slight headache at times.
>
> (Sarah)

It was another two weeks before Sarah was diagnosed with haemolysis, elevated liver enzymes and lowered platelets (HELLP) syndrome. Her blood pressure remained normal and she had no proteinuria. Her condition had 'shown itself' in a preliminary way at 32 weeks but remained hidden when all the test results were negative. She continued to be unwell and on reflection it seems there were very strong signs that all was not well between 32 and 34 weeks. It was fortunate that Sarah was in hospital when she was diagnosed as the condition announced itself with urgency:

> At 34 weeks I was admitted to hospital so that a series of Doppler studies could be done for one of my babies, James. They wanted to do daily measurements every day for a week to make sure there was a good blood supply getting through to him as the sonographer hadn't been able to visualize James's cord very well on my ultrasound and it seemed that he may not have been growing as well as Tim.
>
> (Sarah)

Sarah did not have any of the classic signs of preeclampsia. James was the messenger who initially brought the information that Sarah's pregnancy may be affected by this condition. His suspected poor growth led to Sarah's obstetrician requesting hospital admission. Intra-uterine growth restriction is common with preeclampsia but in itself is just an indication that something is wrong and there are many complex possible contributing factors, especially with a multiple pregnancy.

Smythe (1998) discusses the notion of safety and unsafety in regard to pregnancy. She explores the concept of where the safety or lack of safety lies, suggesting it may be in the darkness, where what is happening is not seen or even imagined (refer to Smythe, Chapter 3). For Sarah, there was unsafety. For her, the unsafety of her preeclampsia was initially 'in the darkness' but revealed itself as the poor fetal growth of one of her babies.

The disease is suddenly very serious

Shortly after admission to hospital Sarah became very unwell:

> I had been in hospital just overnight and had my first lot of blood tests in the morning, then a repeat test about 3 hours later just prior to going for my scan. I had a really awful night. I must have been deteriorating overnight as I had been very restless and couldn't sleep much. I was really, really hot and flushed. I didn't have a fever, someone took my temperature and it was normal but I just felt absolutely dreadful. I was really uncomfortable, so hot that I was getting cold flannels to put on my forehead and felt like I had a temperature of 40°! I didn't think that I was right after a night like that. I knew I shouldn't feel that hot. I had the abdominal pain and back pain during the night as well.

I had a routine blood test that morning and my results were abnormal. My liver enzymes were high and the obstetrician told me that he thought there had been a mistake in the laboratory leading to someone else's results being reported under my name. He ordered a repeat test to be sure, although he did say there was a chance I might have to have the babies that day. I knew that the results were probably right as I was expecting to develop preeclampsia at some stage.

I walked down to the ultrasound department that morning to have my scan and waited for an hour, sitting there with a thumping headache. I hadn't had anything to eat or drink just in case I needed to have an anaesthetic for an emergency delivery and I was feeling really unwell. They were planning to scan my liver as well and the sonographer had just started to do that when the house surgeon came down and said 'Right, We'll take you back in a wheel chair and we'll have to get you ready right now'.

(Sarah)

There is no doubt about Sarah's diagnosis at this stage, although the obstetrician did not at first believe the blood test could be right. There could be a degree of surprise and disbelief when a woman presents atypically with preeclampsia. However, Sarah was certainly at increased risk because of her family history and current pregnancy history. It also seems that she may have had a more realistic awareness of what was happening to her than did her obstetrician. Normal blood pressure may hide preeclampsia and falsely reassure professionals that all is well. However, the blood pressure may become elevated very late in the disease and so much can change so quickly.

The risk of being fooled by semblance

The announcement via the laboratory results was urgent, the condition was revealed and there was no time to wait; Sarah's babies had to be delivered. Prompt delivery resulted in a safe outcome for this woman and her twin sons. What might have happened if she had not been admitted for assessment of fetal wellbeing? Sarah's symptoms could be described as a 'semblance' of several other problems such as a viral infection or cholelithiasis:

I wonder if I should have had some more regular blood tests as had James been growing normally I might not have been diagnosed early enough to have a safe outcome.... My blood pressure had been normal on the day I visited my obstetrician when she admitted me in order to monitor James. I guess if I had interpreted my symptoms as something like a viral infection I might not have been diagnosed had I been at home at that point. I didn't have the classic signs of preeclampsia. I probably would have thought 'I was assessed 2 weeks ago and nothing was wrong, I'm just being paranoid...'.

(Sarah)

A woman at home is perhaps more likely to think 'It's probably nothing serious' so as not to bother anyone or appear to be a worrier. Had Sarah remained at home she may have dismissed her symptoms as she had earlier been investigated in hospital and discharged without any diagnosis.

Not as the textbook describes

For Nadia, a primigravida at 33 weeks, preeclampsia 'announced itself' after her symptoms led to admission to hospital following two days of atypical intermittent pain:

> It was on a Monday, and I was at work. I just had a bit of pain in my chest, but only when I breathed in. It kept going during the day and so I rang the midwife that evening and talked about it and she said well you know it's probably the baby kicking you know, on your ribs and stuff which you know, is pretty normal. Anyway we came to the conclusion it must have been right because, that evening the pain just disappeared, and the next day Tuesday (I took the day off work just because I was feeling tired) I was fine. We went out that night for a Christmas barbeque and everything was fine, then it was about the middle of the night, 2 o'clock in the morning, and I had this back pain between my shoulder blades – constant pain, it didn't go away. So then, on the Wednesday morning I rang the midwife again and said 'something doesn't feel right' and then she said 'Well alright we'll go to the hospital, get us booked in and check it out'. Previously I'd had just a little swelling in my ankles, and a little bit in my hands but nothing major, and my blood pressure was pretty OK.

(Nadia)

Nadia's pain was not the classic epigastric pain experienced with severe preeclampsia. According to Heidegger (1962/1927) a true phenomenon shows itself as it is. But when something shows itself under the guise of what it is not, then we are faced with a semblance, or a 'seeming'. As with the example concerning Lynda, the semblance confounded diagnosis, leading to delayed recognition of preeclampsia.

Nadia describes how the following day she decided to take a day off work as she felt tired. Whilst this is a normal experience in pregnancy, many women recall feeling tired and generally unable to cope prior to the onset of severe preeclampsia. Nadia's pain had settled for 24 hours or more after first appearing. When symptoms hint that something may be wrong and then disappear the condition which may have been 'shown' by the first onset of pain, may seem less likely because of the fleeting or intermittent nature of the symptom. As with Lynda's experience, for Nadia the disease itself remained hidden while progressing silently. The second time the pain occurred Nadia had a sense that all was not well with her pregnancy, and her midwife responded by organizing a prompt specialist assessment.

Urgent announcing

Preeclampsia can announce itself with frightening urgency. In some cases after an apparent improvement or disappearance of symptoms the disease can fulminate and demand an emergency response. For Nadia, who was starting to feel that she was in hospital unnecessarily, the diagnosis of HELLP syndrome left her feeling shocked:

> So they checked me out which took a while because they do your blood tests and everything was fine! I remember the consultant said it was probably gallstones or something like that because the blood tests came back OK. So we thought we might just go have a scan and check the baby out. Anyway of course by about 2 o'clock the pain had gone and I thought 'What are we doing here?' Then it got to about 4 o'clock in the afternoon and I had more blood tests just to double check. The results came back at 5 o'clock showing the platelets were 39! (Normal range 150–450.) The level had been low earlier but nothing to be really concerned about – that was how fast it went. I was feeling better than I had in the morning. I mean – I was like 'Are you sure this is right?' I was really upset.
>
> (Nadia)

Initially, Nadia's symptoms were incorrectly interpreted as discomfort from the baby kicking. Even after initial assessment in hospital the provisional diagnosis was possible gallstones. However, the cause of her symptoms was eventually 'announced' as the phenomenon of preeclampsia by the conclusive laboratory result. This story shows that the blood picture can deteriorate without pain or visible symptoms. This example shows the importance of listening to the woman. It would be easy to dismiss symptoms that are erratic or appear to be resolving but Nadia's midwife had faith in her client's feeling that something was wrong and was prepared to persist until an accurate diagnosis was made. Her concern led to timely intervention for Nadia and her baby Thomas. Delay may have been tragic.

A paradox, which may be very significant for midwives to be aware of, is the fact that most of the women had started to feel better when their preeclampsia was deteriorating to the point where they needed urgent delivery. If a woman has been symptomatic of preeclampsia but her condition has not yet been 'announced' by laboratory testing or other signs, such as hypertension or intra-uterine growth restriction, it may be reassuring for the woman and the midwife when the symptoms improve or disappear. Had Nadia not been admitted for investigations her disappearance of symptoms could have dangerously reassured her and her midwife that all was well.

Unrecognized announcing

Preeclampsia is a disease which progresses unpredictably, and its symptoms are often unexpectedly mild or unusual prior to the point where emergency delivery becomes necessary for the mother's safety. Even on an antenatal ward, staff may not recognize symptoms which announce serious deterioration. Kate remembers experiencing severe pain and breathlessness in the night and telling the nurse who seemed not to understand the significance:

> So the protein had been increasing and my blood pressure had been creeping up, but on the Friday night I had a lot of epigastric pain, pain with breathing and from my point of view I really did not feel good. I suddenly felt sick and threw up and it was all bile. I was having a lot of pain and really uncomfortable and I knew there was something not right. I'd buzzed from the toilet and nobody came. I waited about 20 minutes and I must have crawled back to bed after that and buzzed again. I said to the nurse – "there's something wrong here". I was really uncomfortable with the pain. She didn't do anything about it. I couldn't sleep all night, had a lot of pain, it was shocking. Then the next nurse came on and I must have gone out to the desk and said, "look there's something not right here" or asked to see a doctor or something. They found that my liver and kidneys had inflamed overnight and then they said – "That's it you're going to have your baby now". That was it – I was having an emergency caesarean section that morning. Of course I was crying and I was really upset – I was really terrified for how well Lilly was going to do, I knew it wasn't good for her. Then when I went down to theatre I was so stressed out I was really shaking.
>
> (Kate)

For Kate, the epigastric pain considered to be a classic symptom of severe preeclampsia was not recognized. She experienced severe pain throughout the night and knew that something was not right. The pain, fear and deterioration she experienced during the night culminated in an emergency caesarean in the morning when it was eventually acknowledged that she was very unwell. By the time she went to theatre she was so stressed she was shaking. While this may not be uncommon, for Kate, the previous few hours of pain with no support or reassurance were a 'shocking' prelude to the birth of her baby. As well as the emotional and psychological stress it is possible that the apparent indifference of the nurse or midwife could have led to a very dangerous outcome as Kate's condition was clearly deteriorating rapidly. Even though Kate had been diagnosed with preeclampsia and admitted to hospital for monitoring, her deterioration was dangerously overlooked.

Atypical pain

The pain associated with liver complications in preeclampsia is mentioned in midwifery texts as epigastric (Henderson and McDonald 2004). Several of the participants experienced a different sort of pain, leading me to question the completeness of information in reference books available to midwives, and the consequent advice given to clients. Lynda's initial pain was experienced in her upper back, between the shoulder blades and as she became more unwell in hospital she described her pain in this way:

> I just had that pain in my back but I was having Panadol the whole time I was in there. The pain was kind of between my shoulders and up to my head. It was just like a force, like something was pushing really hard. Yes, it went up to my head, it just felt like pressure basically. I tried to stay as still as I could but it was very uncomfortable, the bed was very uncomfortable and they'd puff up your pillows, and tilt the bed up but there wasn't much relief. If I took Panadol it just kind of took the edge off it – it was mostly just like pressure. I felt restless because I couldn't get comfortable.
>
> (Lynda)

Pain between the shoulder blades is sometimes experienced when there is inflammation in the liver. Lynda never experienced classic epigastric pain at all and the pain that she described could have been attributed to another cause had her condition not been revealed by her hypertension.

For the midwife or doctor who is watching and waiting, trying to keep in step with the woman so that they do not miss a sign which may herald the onset of disease, it can be an anxious time. It is likely that research will uncover a predictive test in the near future (Sunderji *et al.* 2010) which may provide forewarning to the practitioner so that the identified 'at risk' woman may be provided with a level of antenatal surveillance which will keep ahead of the 'showing' and especially the 'announcing'. Until that happens, however, the confusing, hinting, coming-and-going showing of preeclampsia is all there is to initially guide the woman and her practitioner.

Implications for practice

Findings from this study suggest that it is not uncommon that practitioners may miss the warning signs of preeclampsia. Late diagnosis of severe preeclampsia leaves the woman and her practitioner shocked and bewildered. This study highlights that there may be many unrecognized warnings prior to diagnosis as the condition worsens and starts to compromise mother and baby. Preeclampsia is perplexing and unpredictable in its onset and progression. The occurrence of preeclampsia is not restricted to women with recognized risk factors and the vigilant practitioner needs to ensure that no sign or symptom is ignored. Women need to know about preeclampsia. Knowledge may increase anxiety for the pregnant woman but can also be life saving for her and/or her baby. Informed partners and families may be aware of changes unnoticed by the woman, for example facial puffiness, and ensure that a professional opinion is sought in good time. In the near future, predictive tests may alert the practitioner to increased risk and the need for more frequent examination and investigation.

To recap, the women in this study experienced feeling like they had the flu, feeling 'gungy', backache between the shoulder blades, headaches, no energy, uncomfortable at night, backache akin to a urinary infection, vomiting, diarrhoea, restlessness, feeling feverish without a temperature. These are all symptoms easily discounted. A headache is just a headache. Everybody is at risk of getting the flu, or a vomiting bug. Many pregnant women get backache and have trouble sleeping. All of these symptoms can so readily be discounted as 'minor discomforts of pregnancy' with the assumption that they will either go away, or the woman will just have to put up with them.

When oedema, proteinuria and raised blood picture add to the picture, the midwife is more likely to be cued into the possibility of preeclampsia. The salutatory lesson from this research is such 'classic' symptoms may not appear until the disease process is well advanced. While blood tests often dramatically confirmed preeclampsia, there first needs to be a reason for such tests to be ordered. The classic epigastric pain was only described by one woman in this study. 'Epigastric' is not a word commonly used in everyday language. It is unlikely a woman would even know to describe a pain by such a word, even though that is the word that textbooks would have the health professional attuned to in terms of a diagnosis of preeclampsia.

Smythe (2000) refers to the spirit of safe practice that is always open to possibilities. The findings of this study suggest that midwives need always to be asking themselves 'could this be preeclampsia?' Even if the symptoms seem to be 'ordinary', the question needs to be kept in mind. More than that, a listening attitude to practice will draw forth words from the woman that describe a feeling of unwellness that is almost indescribable. It does not fit any known pattern. While the woman might say she has a headache, or feels like she has the flu, she says it in a tone that suggests it is more than that, but she is not sure what to call this dramatic (or creeping) change in her wellbeing.

Further, the woman herself, and her family need to know that there is a disease called preeclampsia that can develop dramatically. They are the people who are 'there' to notice and respond. Herein lies the tension of practice: to frighten women and have them anxious about every minor discomfort, or to prepare them so they may access prompt life-saving treatment. Every woman has the right to know about the possibility of preeclampsia, and every midwife and doctor has the responsibility to be watching closely; even when there is little to suggest a problem. Of the eight women in this study, one baby died because of preeclampsia and extreme prematurity. All of these women had their health severely compromised, and their babies were significantly at risk. By considering each woman's individual risk profile, weighing up the likelihood of preeclampsia, and responding appropriately to the 'showing' it is less likely that the abnormal will be normalized, delaying diagnosis and increasing risk.

Conclusion

The knowledge and support of practitioners can contribute positively to women's safety and experience of preeclampsia. Whilst it is likely that screening tests to enable safe and timely diagnosis will soon be available, in the meantime, practitioners who work with women in a relationship based on trust and openness may be the most able to recognize preeclampsia as it shows itself and support the women through the inevitable intervention and holistic recovery. The consequences of full-blown preeclampsia are devastating. We have a mandate to do all we can to keep women safe. This is not a disease that can be ignored. It needs to be at the forefront of everyone's minds.

References

Baker P.N. and Kingdom J.C.P. (eds) (2004) *Pre-eclampsia Current Perspectives on Management*. Parthenon: London.

Caelli K. (2001) Engaging with phenomenology: Is it more of a challenge than it needs to be? *Qualitative Health Research* 11 (2), 271–281.

Cowan J. (1997) Wendy's Story. *New Zealand College of Midwives Journal* 16, 20–23.

Crotty M. (1998) *The Foundations of Social Research*. Allen and Unwin: NSW.

Duley L., Meher S. and Abalos E. (2006) Management of Preeclampsia. *BMJ* 332, 463–468.

Gadamer H. G. (1982/1960) *Truth and Method* (Barden, G. and Cumming, J., trans). Crossroads: New York.

Heidegger M. (1962/1927) *Being and Time* (Macquarie, J. and Robinson, E., trans.). Basil Blackwell Ltd: Oxford.

Henderson C. and McDonald S. (eds). (2004) *Mayes Midwifery. A Textbook for Midwives*. (13th edn). Bailliere Tindall: Edinburgh.

Kleiman S. (2004) Phenomenology: to wonder and search for meanings. *Nurse Researcher* 11 (4), 7–19.

Matthys L.A., Coppage K.H., Lambers D.S., Barton J.R. and Sibai B.M. (2004) Delayed postpartum preeclampsia: An experience of 151 cases. *American Journal of Obstetrics and Gynecology* 190 (5), 1464–1466.

Redman C.W. and Sargent I.L. (2005) Latest advances in understanding preeclampsia, *Science* 303, 1592–1594.

The SCOPE Study. http://www.scopestudy.net [Accessed 31 January 2010].

Serenius F., Ewald U., Faroogi A., Holmgren P-A., Hakansson S. and Sedin G. (2004) Short term outcome after active perinatal management at 23–25 weeks of gestation. A study from two Swedish tertiary care centres. Part 1: maternal and obstetric factors. *Acta Paediatrica* 93 (7), 945–953.

Smythe E. A. (1998) 'Being safe' in childbirth: A hermeneutic interpretation of the narratives of women and practitioners. *Unpublished PhD thesis*, Massey University: Palmerston North, New Zealand.

Smythe E. (2000) 'Being safe' in childbirth: what does it mean? A phenomenological/ hermeneutic approach, *New Zealand College of Midwives Journal* 22, 18–21.

Sunderji S., Gaziano E., Wothe D., Rogers C. L., Sibai B., Karumanchi S. A. and Hodges-Savola C. (2010) Automated assays for sVEGF R1 and PlGF as an aid in the diagnosis of preterm preeclampsia: a prospective clinical study. *Am J Obstet Gynecol* (serial online). 202 (1): 40e1–7. Available from MEDLINE: Ipswich, MA. [Accessed 30 January 2010].

van Manen M. (1990) *Researching Lived Experience: Human Science for an Action Sensitive Pedagogy.* State University of New York Press: London, Ontario.

Weintraub S. (2003) *Charlotte and Lionel A Rothschild Love Story.* The Free Press: New York.

7 The meaning of giving birth from a long-term perspective for childbearing women

Ingela Lundgren

Introduction

My initial research into childbirth stemmed from my experiences as a midwife (Lundgren 2002). I was astonished at how differently experiences of childbirth were expressed. Some women radiated harmony and happiness and told me that the experience had had a great positive influence on them. Simply by looking at them I could see that giving birth had been empowering and strengthening. However, I have also encountered women who told me that giving birth was the worst experience in their life; a terrifying engagement with fear of death, which they hoped they would never experience again. These encounters inspired me to study childbirth experiences and, specifically, the meaning of giving birth for the lives of women. The meaning of events for people's lives is best explored using a phenomenological method. In phenomenology the focus lies in the description of a phenomenon, which is an object as a subject experiences it. An object could, for example, be childbirth experiences. From a phenomenological perspective it is not possible to describe an object, such as childbirth experiences, without reference to the subjects. In the case of the studies presented in this chapter, this is the women who took part. However, it is not possible to search for a definitive meaning, since people always live in relation to time and space (Merleau-Ponty 1995). Meaning is never fixed nor static, but contextual and historical (Dahlberg *et al.* 2008). This means that the chronological moment when the studies in this chapter were undertaken and the context they took place in, are formative for the phenomenon of women's meaning of giving birth from a long-term perspective. The section below on methodology explores this in more detail.

Background

Giving birth is a life event (Larkin *et al.* 2009, Bondas 2005), with an opportunity for the woman to gain an understanding of her strengths, and connection with other women (Callister 2004). In recent years, giving birth has been established as an event that can be perceived as traumatic

(Sawyer and Ayers 2009). A transformative experience implies victories and strength, healing, and short- and long-term outcomes (Kennedy *et al.* 2004). A traumatic birth experience could have a long lasting effect on the woman's health and well-being (Beck 2006). The most important factor for a positive childbirth experience for the birthing woman is support (Hodnett *et al.* 2007), and much research describes the significance of the midwife's support to the woman (Hunter 2002, Bowers 2002). Not being supportive can be related to uncaring behaviours, and undesired interactions (Halldorsdottir and Karlsdottir 1996).

The results of my studies show that the relationship between the midwife and the birthing woman may be conceptualized under the heading 'releasing and relieving encounters'. For the woman, it is an encounter with herself as well as with the midwife. The encounter implies stillness as well as change, which for the midwife equals being both 'anchored' and a 'companion' (Lundgren 2002). As Simkin (1991) has shown, birth experiences are of importance to women years after the event has taken place. According to Callister (2004), by listening to women and their birth stories health professionals can help women to integrate a major event in their lives.

However, most studies in this area are conducted in the first few days and weeks following birth (Lundgren *et al.* 2009). In this chapter I will describe the results from three phenomenological studies that took a longer-term perspective, namely one to four years after birth (Lundgren 2005, Lundgren 2010, Nilsson *et al.* 2010).

Methodology

All three studies used a phenomenological method, based on a lifeworld approach (Dahlberg *et al.* 2008; also see Chapter 2). The purpose of phenomenological research is to describe phenomena as they are lived and experienced by individuals. Based on the work of the philosophers Husserl (1979) and Merleau-Ponty (1995), lifeworld research seeks the patterns, structures and principles of the meaning of experiences, as well as unique experiences. Openness is central for lifeworld research. In line with Gadamer's (1995) concept of scientific openness, it is described as a wish to see and understand something in a new way. Lifeworld research is governed by some general principles. The data analysis is described as a movement between the whole – to the parts – and back to the whole. During analysis, the researcher moves from understanding the interview text as a whole, through understanding the single meaning units of the text, to a new whole, in which the essential meaning of the phenomenon is illuminated (Dahlberg *et al.* 2008).

Phenomenological studies must always be interpreted in relation to their context and time, and thus can never be understood as presenting universal claims. However, the fact that the results are contextual does not imply that they would be inapplicable and have no meaning in other contexts.

Application of the results to new contexts entails an open-ended process of understanding, which is also depicted in the metaphor of the hermeneutic circle (Heidegger 1998/1927). Results from phenomenological research in childbirth can be understood as yielding a deeper understanding of the similarities and the common structure of women's experiences by describing the essential structure, without ignoring the uniqueness of the individuals involved.

Context and method

All three studies were conducted in Sweden (Lundgren 2005, Nilsson *et al.* 2010, Lundgren 2010). Swedish maternity care is funded by taxes, and is free at the point of use. Almost all births take place in a hospital-based maternity unit. Professional midwives are responsible for the care of women with normal pregnancies and births. An obstetrician takes over the responsibility if there are complications or risk factors during the pregnancy or the birth. Home birth is not included in public health care, and today, there are no birth centres. A study by Hildingsson *et al.* (2003) showed that 8 per cent of a sample of Swedish women expressed an interest in birth centre care when these women were asked in early pregnancy, and at two months and one year after birth. Therefore, if women in Sweden were offered a free choice of place of birth, the 20 largest hospitals would need to have a birth centre. The same study by Hildingsson *et al.* (2003) showed that 1 per cent of the women expressed an interest in giving birth at home.

The context for the first study was a birth centre (Lundgren 2005). The phenomenon of focus was women's experiences of childbirth two years after the birth. Birth centres provide midwifery-led care, continuity of care, a home-like environment, and restrictions on the use of medical technology (Kirkham 2003). If complications occur, the women are transferred to standard care in hospital. At the time of the study, there were three birth centres in Sweden (these are all now closed). The birth centre in the study was situated alongside a hospital and had two delivery rooms and some family rooms for postnatal care. Antenatal care was not provided at the birth centre; instead, a preparatory visit before the delivery was integrated in the service. However, as a project in 1996–1997, when the women in this study gave birth, women were given an opportunity to receive antenatal care at the unit.

With regards to the second study, professional maternity care at home is not included in public healthcare provision in Sweden (Lundgren 2010). The official statistics do not separate planned and unplanned home births. By studying the Swedish Medical Birth Register, 1992–2004, Hildingsson *et al.* (2006) found that the rate for planned home birth was less than one in a thousand. Only a small number of midwives conduct home births and they take place in only a limited number of areas in Sweden. A few counties pay private midwives, assisting women at home, if the woman meets certain medical criteria (Stockholms läns landsting (Textbook for Midwives) 2002). The study explored women's experiences of giving birth and making decisions about whether to give birth at home. The women in this study resided in a county that did not provide home birth opportunities.

The context for the third study was a special clinic for women with fear of childbirth (Nilsson *et al.* 2010). The aim of this study was to uncover the meanings of previous experiences of childbirth in pregnant women who had intense fear of childbirth. In Swedish samples, 6 to 10 per cent of pregnant women reported such fear, defined as having a clear impact on their everyday life, very negative feelings when pregnant, and thinking about delivery during the pregnancy, or having to undergo counselling because of their fear (Areskog *et al.* 1981, Waldenström *et al.* 2006). In most Swedish hospitals, treatment for fear of childbirth is provided by specially trained midwives, called 'Aurora teams'. Women who present with signs of intense fear of childbirth are referred by maternity center midwives or physicians. After appraisal by the team, the woman can attend two or three counselling sessions with a midwife, although additional appointments can be offered as necessary.

Participants

The study based in the birth centre comprised interviews with ten women who intended to have a birth centre birth while they were pregnant. Five of these were multiparous and five primiparous (Lundgren 2005). Seven of the women actually gave birth in the birth centre. Two primiparous women were transferred to the standard delivery ward during delivery because of prolonged labour. One of the multiparous women did not give birth at the birth centre because of breech presentation. The women were interviewed on one occasion, two years after the birth.

Seven women were recruited for the study about giving birth and making decisions about whether to give birth at home. These participants included one primiparous woman and six who were multiparous (Lundgren 2010). All of these women had been actively searching for professional support for a home birth. Four of the women, all multiparous, ended up giving birth at home without the professional assistance of a midwife. Three of these women had previously given birth at home with the professional assistance of a midwife, and one of them had given birth at hospital. The other women (*n*=3) gave birth in a hospital, and all of them had a doula as extra support during the birth. Data were collected by interviews during 2007, one to three years after their previous births. Women were recruited through an organization in Gothenburg, Sweden (födelsehuset; www.fodelsehuset.se) supporting women's opportunity to have different forms of care during childbirth.

Nine multiparous women participated in the study about previous experiences of birth in women with intense fear of childbirth (Nilsson *et al.*

2010). At the time of interview, all the women were pregnant with their second child (18 to 39 gestational weeks). All women had had a self-defined negative birth experience. Four of the women had had a normal vaginal birth, two had had a vacuum extraction, and three an emergency caesarean section. All except one were planning for a vaginal birth in their forthcoming birth. Data were gathered in 2006–2007 through interviews with pregnant women one to four years after their previous birth.

Analysis

For each study, the data analysis was conducted following the description of Dahlberg *et al.* (2008; refer also to Chapter 2). The interviews were transcribed verbatim and analysed by the interviewer. Each interview was first read to bring out a sense of the whole and, after that, meaning units were marked. Meaning units are smaller segments of the text, which are of relevance for the studied phenomenon (Giorgi 1997). The meaning of the text was organized into different clusters by 'unpacking' the meaning of the text and relating the meaning units to each other. In the final operation, the essential structure of the investigated phenomenon, a description of what has been revealed, was formulated. The essential structure was further explained by its constituents, namely the particulars and meanings that constitute the actual essence.

A synthesis of the three studies (Lundgren 2005, Lundgren 2010, Nilsson *et al.* 2010) will now be presented. The analysis is a secondary analysis (Heaton 2004, Thorne 1994) using original data from the studies. One suggestion for data analysis, according to Heaton (2004), is to follow the same qualitative method as the original studies. In the analysis of the three studies, the overall question was what meaning components are central for women's experiences of childbirth from a long-term perspective. The themes that emerged from the synthesis are presented in this chapter.

Ethical considerations

According to Swedish law at the time of the study by Nilsson *et al.* (2010) and Lundgren (2010), ethical approval was not required for research studies that did not pose a physical or mental risk to the informants (Swedish Health Care Act 2003, p. 460). Nevertheless, the Regional Ethics Board was consulted about the studies and we received written verification that no formal permission was required. Ethical approval and permission to undertake the study by Lundgren (2005) was obtained from the Regional Ethics Board. Permission to conduct and audio-tape the interviews was obtained in writing from each participant and the participants were assured both verbally and in writing that all information would be treated confidentially. The information to the potential participants as well as the informed consent form was designed to reflect the basic principles decided by the

Regional Ethics Board. In all studies women were given an opportunity to talk to the interviewer and ask further questions on completion of the interviews. The women could also be referred to a physician, midwife or psychologist if necessary.

Secondary analysis is a research strategy which makes use of pre-existing research data for the purpose of investigating new questions or verifying previous studies. The re-use of data for purposes other than which it was collected (whether this is by the same researchers, who were involved in the primary research or by other researchers) raises a number of ethical and legal issues. For instance, should the researcher obtain informed consent for a secondary analysis, and if so, when would be the best time for this (Heaton 2004)? In this study the same researcher as in the original studies was involved. Furthermore, the new research question, the meaning of giving birth from a long-term perspective for childbearing women is very closely related to the primary research question(s).

Findings

Based on the results from the secondary analysis three themes emerged: 'strengthening and disempowering', 'being a subject and an object' and 'supportive and not supportive'. Giving birth has meaning for the women in relation to their own development, and to the changes that happen to them after birth. This process can be experienced as 'strengthening' for some, but as 'disempowering' for others. Furthermore, the meaning of giving birth is related to the woman's own role during the birth. Being 'a subject' means to actively participate during birth. However, some women could also experience a lack of participation in the birth experience and instead became 'an object' for others. Finally, the meaning of giving birth for childbearing women can be related to professional behaviours, in particular that midwives, who can be experienced as 'supportive' or 'not supportive'.

Strengthening and disempowering

The birth centre study illuminated the fact that giving birth can be experienced as an empowering and life-changing experience for women. The participants expressed a strengthening of self-confidence, and trust in their own capacity. They were proud of their capacity to give birth:

> I see the delivery as a milestone that, in a way, has helped me to grow as a human being, and you don't forget that, but this has just made me stronger, and more vulnerable too, although I don't know how to explain it…it outweighs the strength you get…so if you are more vulnerable you can manage it much better.
>
> (Participant 1)

Some of the women described how they became more aware of their own feelings and wishes following childbirth, and how they were now able to ask for help if they needed it. This was expressed as a strengthening of self-understanding:

> I think I am a person who can camouflage myself and have an ability to pretend. I should have made it clearer…but I have learnt to speak out my opinion so I feel it is positive anyway and nothing I would have had undone…you learn so much from everything you experience, so I probably have learned a little about myself that I reacted in a way I hadn't expected but at the same time you feel that nothing anyway could be harder than this… you feel strong too.
>
> (Participant 5)

Birth as strengthening was also expressed by women who wanted a home birth. They described the birth with words such as 'power', 'force' and 'wonder'. Childbirth was experienced as thrilling and the women described how they had matured through the process. They had encountered themselves during the birth. They were proud about giving birth, and expressed respect for themselves. Birth was seen as something empowering and strengthening which had importance for bonding between the mother and child:

> It was exciting. I hardly ate or slept. It lasted for 2 weeks. And my sister told me I was totally speeded when she talked to me by telephone. I'm so happy for having this experience. For us it was really important because in early pregnancy we didn't want this child. It meant everything. I have never been so in love in my whole life as I became in him.
>
> (Participant 15)

Previous birth experiences for the women who had intense fear of childbirth were described as disempowering. Their experiences were associated with fear, loneliness, a lack of faith in their ability to give birth and diminished trust in maternity care:

> It was sort of a long black hole. It felt like no let-up, just endless, endless pain. Nothing to hold on to…. The feeling in my chest of becoming totally empty…. It's that feeling… drained of strength and energy and zest for life.
>
> (Participant 18)

These women expressed dread towards their forthcoming birth and were afraid of a repetition of their previous experience. For some of the women this fear had lingered unnoticed until they became pregnant again:

> I was of course aware that I found it hard but I don't think I had quite taken it in emotionally until now when I am pregnant again.... I've realized that with that experience in my mental baggage I can't just go there and assume that I will give birth just like that [snapping her fingers].
>
> (Participant 19)

Similar accounts were given by women who wanted a home birth. All women who gave birth at home without professional assistance had had a previous negative birth at hospital. Following this, the women reported that they were fearful, depressed and sad. They described how they attempted to internalize these feelings by finding out what had happened during the birth and by receiving professional support from midwives, physicians and psychologists:

> I was very sad for a long time after that birth and it was hard for other people to understand. My mother-in-law and my mother and everybody thought everything went well and I had a healthy baby. You didn't have to have a caesarean or anything so you should be pleased.
>
> (Participant 12)

A disempowering experience of birth is contrasted with brief moments that made sense for women with intense fear of childbirth:

> It [the bearing down] was the best phase of the whole delivery because then something was happening... it was an act that I could do myself.
>
> (Participant 13)

A good experience was described as being present in the moment and in oneself. However, for women with traumatic birth memories these moments did not remain a part of the women's birth experience.

Being a subject and an object

Being a subject meant to actively participate during the birth. This was described as 'going with the flow and at the same time taking command of themselves'. These descriptions were provided by women who gave birth at the birth centre. Being a subject meant that women were guided by their bodily signals:

> Well, it was so powerful. It was unlike anything else. As in very bad weather, such as a very heavy thunderstorm, a snowstorm or something. You can't control it. Something was happening regardless of what you do. I must say it's very, very groovy.
>
> (Participant 4)

Trust in themselves, their capacity to give birth, and their body were crucial for being a 'subject'. At the same time as the women were letting the process of childbirth be in charge, they wanted to take command of themselves: to be in control in order not to lose themselves and their participation in the experience of childbirth:

> You get concentrated when the pain comes and feel that the pain is developing something... to follow and see the connection in relation to the opening. During my last delivery, it was more like... no I don't want this. But now I was no longer a victim. Instead, I was more co-operative and more in control of myself, you may say.
>
> (Participant 6)

Similar descriptions were given by women who wanted to give birth at home. They held an inner image of birth characterized by trust and their own capacity to give birth and actively participate. Personal responsibility was related to an opportunity to calmly enter the process of birth. If this was possible, the women could concentrate on the birth process without being disturbed by external events. They entered their own world and followed the process of birth, which could be described as mentally encountering the birth. This process was described by a woman who gave birth at home:

> I have a strong 'body knowledge' and I can feel what is happening in my body...it was a fantastic experience... I felt when the head was crowning... and after that it was a break...and my husband in astonishment said... the baby's eyebrow and nose are moving... he could see her face...And after the next contraction the whole head was out and after the next – the whole baby. First, I was worried because she was so quiet but her skin color was fine. She was so quiet because the birth was not disturbed. It was a very calm birth.
>
> (Participant 13)

However, some of the women considered the responsibilities of giving birth at home without professional assistance were too heavy. These women wanted a midwife to confirm the process of birth. To have entered into the process of birth and simultaneously feel a need to track the stages of labour was problematic:

> And I became a little worried because I couldn't recognize where I was in the process. And I blamed the fact that I didn't have a midwife who could check where I was.
>
> (Participant 16)

Women with intense fear of childbirth felt that they had not actively participated during their previous birth. Instead they felt themselves to be 'beside' or 'outside' the experience. The women felt that they were not entirely present in themselves, in the here and now, in the room and/or in relation to other people. This can be related to being 'an object':

> I was more or less an object, not a human being but something they had to get something out of, nobody told me anything, nobody said a word, no explanations nor any kind of information whatsoever.
>
> (Participant 20)

Further, these women considered that they were not physically able or allowed to participate in the experience of childbirth. It was an experience that they did not fully understand, and that 'just happened' to their bodies. They expressed shock and loneliness and a lack of understanding as to why they were there. The women felt as if they had no place there, that they were unable to take their place:

> I felt so suppressed that in normal cases I would have yelled at someone who treated me like that … It felt as if everything was locked inside me, I was almost crouching in a corner. Like, excuse me for being here. I was hoping to give birth to a child today, is that okay? … I didn't recognize myself.
>
> (Participant 20)

Supportive and not supportive

The study from the birth centre illuminated how support and help from the midwife were central for the women's ability to go with the flow and take command of themselves. Participants appeared to believe that the midwife's primary role was to see the woman and her needs, to support the woman's ability to follow the phases of childbirth, and to be confident in the woman's capacity to give birth:

> Well, they just kept… I felt that they were present for us and were there for us but that they didn't…they continuously observed the delivery and how the land lay. So they didn't just rush in and say 'Now you are going to give birth – just calmly lean back'…and so on…and 'Hi there' and give good advice…Instead they were very sensitive and I was able to be myself and could show all sides of myself and was still believed in, so to speak.
>
> (Participant 2)

Giving birth caused feelings of helplessness if the labour was not progressing, when contractions and the pain were not in harmony, and when women were unable to influence their situation:

I had lost focus and it was just continuing and continuing... and I had reached all my boundaries, physically as well as mentally, I was just blubbering and wanted to die. I was in a cul-de-sac......I was sort of locked in a cave and I couldn't get through anywhere.

(Participant 1)

In order to continue the process of childbirth, women in this situation needed help from the midwife. At this point, she needed to intervene, and such interventions tended to create strong feelings of relief even if the women had previously expected a natural birth without medical interventions:

I can't get through anywhere, I'm totally deadlocked and at this moment of great despair it seemed that a kind of 'laser elevator' came down and that the doors opened, and 'Welcome! Step inside and you will be delivered' ... there is a way out.

(Participant 2)

Help with the process of childbirth was also central for women with an intense fear of childbirth. They reported that they did not receive information about the progress of the birth or the state of the baby. Even if the midwife was present, she did not provide support. Sometimes, the only focus seemed to be on practical and technical aspects. In the following case, the midwife failed to provide the woman with the necessary support, such as commitment and encouragement:

And she was very cold and very hard and didn't touch me in any way. She was sitting on the floor looking at me, she sort of couldn't, she didn't talk to me properly and wasn't a gentle kind of person. I sort of felt that I couldn't choose myself; I wanted somebody to guide me.... I didn't understand anything about all that, thought it was really weird... it was as if she didn't believe that I was in pain.

(Participant 21)

Similar experiences of their previous labours were described by some of the women who wanted a home birth. They had experienced superiority and authority from non-supportive midwives. Their earlier births were described as an event in which they felt totally alienated from themselves and the midwife. Indeed, this extended to a feeling that the midwife was afraid of her, and of the birth. In the following quote, this led to the woman's inability to communicate with her midwife or her husband:

I needed help and my husband knew I was afraid. It was not possible to communicate with me, it didn't work out. The midwife didn't understand the situation.

(Participant 17)

Women with fear of childbirth had brief moments that made sense during the birth when midwives tried to improve a desperate situation; reassured the woman, and created positive energy for her. In some cases, women talked about individual midwives whose support and help was exactly what the women wanted, who was 'perfectly in tune' and thus provided the right kind of support:

> I just thought how wonderful that you are coming back. Somebody I can trust.... Yes, I suppose I got some kind of power then so now I'll do as she says, I can do anything now.... So then I stood up, I stood up in the bed.
>
> (Participant 22)

Women who wanted to give birth at home without receiving any professional assistance did talk about individual midwives and physicians who were supportive. In contrast, as a group midwives and obstetricians were felt to be insecure and unsupportive, and this was seen as indicative of the whole system:

> I felt that she had wanted to help me but her professional duties told her not to do home births. She carefully informed me about this condition. I was happy to finally get some help. With my first child I didn't dare to ask. I was afraid because they were so critical. I was happy to meet her but I appreciated her as a person and not as a healthcare representative.
>
> (Participant 16)

Women who wanted a home birth but who, in the end, decided to give birth in hospital described the hospital birth as being 'as good as it could be'. They all had a doula present during the birth. They experienced the care as meeting their needs, especially when having a midwife who had a positive attitude towards their special needs. In the following case, the women even felt that the hospital staff learned something from her 'unusual hospital birth':

> We had a doula. She was really the person who protected us and was my spokesperson. They left us pretty much alone. Then a new midwife came and she had worked at a birth centre and she was very calm and there were no problems. She used the Pinard stethoscope. The hospital staff thought it was an unusual hospital birth. They were very respectful.
>
> (Participant 26)

Discussion

The strength of a phenomenological study is the opportunity to understand a phenomenon from the participant's perspective. The three studies reported here are from different contexts. Two of them include experiences from women who gave birth in a range of settings, including on a standard delivery ward in hospital, at home, and in a birth centre. The third study was about pregnant women with an intense fear of childbirth, who described their previous negative birth experience. One limitation of the synthesis presented in this chapter might therefore be that many of the women included did not have similar experiences to most childbearing women in Sweden, almost all of whom choose to give birth in hospital. Another limitation of the studies is that qualitative research is contextual and must be related to time and place (see Introduction).

Similar findings emerged from the three studies, despite their different contexts. They illuminated that, from a long-term perspective, giving birth can be experienced as both 'strengthening' and/or 'disempowering'. Further, giving birth can be related to both 'being a subject' and an 'object'. 'Supportive' and 'unsupportive' care from professionals, in particular midwives, is important to the meanings women ascribe to their birth experience.

The themes described the long-term meanings of childbirth for women in a rather polarized way. These main themes can be seen as two sides of the same coin. Women who gave birth at the birth centre and at home mainly describe birth as a strengthening experience. They felt that they acted as a subject and had a supportive midwife, even if being an object and having a non-supportive midwife was also a part of their experience. Women with a fear of childbirth described their previous birth as a disempowering experience. Even if they experienced brief moments of being a subject and receiving support, these moments did not remain a part of their birth experience; instead their lingered memories were of being objects for others and not receiving support.

A secondary analysis has a potential to compare differences across the data and the context (Heaton 2004). There is a need to understand the influence of different birth environments on women's childbirth experiences (Kirkham 2003). However, the specific data from this study are particular to the women included, and the time at which the data was collected. It is not possible to say from this study that giving birth at home and at a birth centre is inevitably more strengthening than giving birth in other contexts. Studies of different settings do suggest that the meanings women attribute to giving birth are related to the context, with more positive accounts from non-hospital settings (Kirkham 2003, Milan 2003, Hodnett *et al.* 2005). However, experiences of strengthening and empowering have also been reported in connection to unmedicated hospital births (Hardin and Buckner 2004). This question should be further studied. This could be done by a quantitative study measuring childbirth experiences in relation to strengthening/disempowering factors, and by a qualitative study focusing on the phenomenon of a strengthening or disempowering childbirth experience.

A strengthening experience could be equated with Maslow's (1979) concept of 'peak experience', which is characterized by joyous and exciting moments in life, involving sudden feelings of intense happiness and well-being, wonder and awe, and also possibly involving an awareness of transcendental unity or knowledge of higher truth. Lahood (2007) claims that traditional birth in different cultures is connected to experiences of 'non-ordinary states of consciousness', 'religious', or 'peak'. Many women find strength and wisdom by passing through these states in labour. In the synthesized data above, women who wanted a home birth described an elevated mood and heightened awareness of the baby, which for one woman lasted up to 14 days after birth. According to the women, this altered state of mind was important in the bonding between the woman and her child. This kind of phenomenon is also noted by Brudal (1980), who states that having a child represents a regressive shift in a person's level of functioning. Such a 'regression in the service of reproduction' brings with it possibilities for growth, but also for extensive pathological regression.

The study about previous birth experiences in women with intense fear of childbirth showed that giving birth was 'disempowering' for the participants. The essence of this was similar to that found in the accounts of multiparous women who wanted a home birth. Some of these women gave birth at home without professional assistance because they could not receive any help.

For women with an intense fear of childbirth the birth experience was etched in their mind and has left scars in the shape of fear, anxiety, loneliness, anger and grief as well as a lack of faith in their own ability to give birth and diminished trust in maternity care. These results have similarities with women's self-defined experience of birth trauma (Beck 2004a, Thomson and Downe 2008). In the study by Thomson and Downe (2008), being isolated and alienated from the birth events is similar to the experience of not being present, as well as to the out-of-body experience described by Beck (2004b). Further, the findings can be related to post-traumatic stress (PTS) and post-traumatic stress disorder (PTSD) after childbirth (Ayers 2007, Beck 2004b, also refer to Beck, Chapter 11). Creedy *et al.* (2000) and Soet *et al.* (2003) claim that a high level of obstetric intervention as well as dissatisfaction with medical personnel during birth are important factors in women's experiences of birth trauma. Distrust towards medical professionals is also expressed by women who want an unassisted birth at home (Lynch 2007, Nolan 2008). For the studies in this synthesis, the same finding of distrust towards medical professionals was described both by women who wanted a homebirth and who decided to give birth without professional assistance, and by women with an intense fear of childbirth. The association between negative experiences of birth and forthcoming childbearing should be further studied. Could one solution be seeking help for their fear and another to avoid the healthcare system and give birth without the professional assistance of a midwife?

The meaning of giving birth was also related to the woman's own role during the birth. Being 'a subject' means to actively participate. The relationship with the midwife was of importance for the women's ability to be a subject. As other authors have noted, positive relations between the midwife and the women are characterized by partnerships of equality (Pairman 2006) and sharing of responsibility (Lundgren 2004). Trust and respect (Kennedy 1995, Page 2003) and reciprocity over time (Fleming 1998, Stevens 2003) are of importance. According to Olafsdottir (2006) an effective relationship in this context has a potential for sharing of information, joint decision making and empowerment for both women and midwives. By being an anchored companion the midwife can help the woman to face the unknown without fear, to be attentive to the birthing process, to feel trust in her own body, and to trust her own ability (Lundgren 2002). The challenge for midwives is to encourage the woman to be 'fully there' in this transition and special state of mind, but not to pass the limits of her capacity (Lundgren 2002).

Some women in the study also experienced a sense of non-participation, and of becoming an 'object' for others. Women with an intense fear of childbirth experienced a physical inability to participate, and/or a lack of permission to do so from the staff. Instead they felt that it was impossible to actively participate or understand, and that things 'just happened' to their bodies. Further, they lacked a relationship with the midwife that was characterized by partnership, equality, trust and respect, and sharing of responsibility as mentioned above. Similar descriptions of earlier births were expressed by multiparous women who wanted a home birth.

The philosopher Merleau-Ponty (1995) introduced the concept of the 'subjective body'. He sought to surpass the problem of the old Cartesian dichotomy of body/soul. According to Merleau-Ponty (1995) one's own living body is not to be understood as a thing, but instead it is the subject and performer of all actions. This means that a human being does not 'have' a body, but instead 'is' her/his body. A person cannot step outside the body, as it is experienced from the inside as well as from the outside simultaneously (Dahlberg *et al.* 2008). The body is both a quasi-object (something that can be observed as if it were a thing), yet at the same time it is *me*, it is the very medium through which there can be other objects for me at all. The body is, therefore, a special kind of 'thing', which I cannot really 'objectively observe'. In contrast to this approach, it can be argued that the science of medicine, focusing only on the 'body' side of the Cartesian split, has during the course of the last few centuries sedimented a notion of the body that most Western cultures seem to subscribe to unproblematically. This notion states that the body is first and foremost a conglomerate of physiological processes, bones, tissues, fluids and cells. This body may be prodded and examined, both inside and out. As a consequence of this attitude, the body is thought to be a kind of machine, mechanized and obedient to the rules of physics, while the human soul is something different from the body (Bullington 1999). However, as the women in this synthesis demonstrate, this so-called objective body does not equal the body, which is the vehicle for each individual's existence, the lived body (Bullington 1999). The phenomenon of being subject and object demonstrate these two diametrically opposed interpretations of the meaning of the body, specifically in the context of childbirth.

Conclusion and practical implications

The three studies reported here show that childbirth experiences are still of importance to women, up to four years after the birth itself. Similar findings emerge from the three studies, despite their different contexts. They show that, from a long-term perspective, giving birth can be experienced as both 'strengthening' and/or 'disempowering'. Furthermore, giving birth can be related to both 'being a subject' and an 'object'. 'Supportive' and 'unsupportive' care from professionals, in particular midwives, is important to the meanings women ascribe to their birth experience.

The conclusion is that childbirth experience has a potential to strengthen self-confidence and trust in others or on the contrary, it can lead to internalizations of failure or distrust. Maternity care should be organized in a way that encourages supportive relationships between midwives and women. Women's own participation should be enabled so that they can become an active subject in the process, and not just an object for others to attend to.

References

Areskog B., Uddenberg N. and Kjessler B. (1981) Fear of childbirth in late pregnancy. *Gynecologic and Obstetric Investigation* 12, 262–266.

Ayers S. (2007) Thoughts and emotions during traumatic birth: A qualitative study. *Birth* 34, 253–263.

Beck C.T. (2004a) Birth trauma: In the eye of the beholder. *Nursing Research* 53, 28–35.

Beck C.T. (2004b) Post-traumatic stress disorder due to childbirth. *Nursing Research* 53, 216–224.

Beck C.T. (2006) Pentadic cartiography: Mapping birth trauma narratives. *Qualitative Health Research* 16 (4), 453–466.

Bondas T. (2005) To be with child: a heuristic synthesis in maternal care. In: *Trends in Midwifery Research* (ed. R. Balin), 119–136. Nova Science: New York.

Bowers B.B. (2002) Mothers experiences of labour support: Exploration of qualitative research. *Journal of Obstetric, Gynecologic and Neonatal Nursing* 31, 742–752.

Brudal L. (1980) Sexuelle samlivsproblemer eg fodsel (Sexual marital problems and childbirth). *Nordisk Psykologi* 32, 42–54.

Bullington J. (1999) *The Mysterious Life of the Body: A New Look at Psychosomatics.* (Doctoral dissertation) Linköping University. Almqvist & Wiksell International: Stockholm.

Callister L.C. (2004) Making meaning: women's birth narratives. *Journal of Obstetric, Gynecologic and Neonatal Nursing* 33, 508–518.

Creedy D., Shochet I. and Horsfall J. (2000) Childbirth and the development of acute trauma symptoms: Incidence and contributing factors. *Birth* 27, 104–111.

Dahlberg K., Dahlberg H. and Nyström M. (2008) *Reflective Lifeworld Research.* Studentlitteratur: Lund.

Fleming V.E. (1998) Women-with-midwives-with-women: a model of interdependence. *Midwifery* 14, 137–143.

Gadamer H.G. (1995) *Truth and Method.* The Continuum Publishing Company: New York.

Giorgi A. (1997) The theory, practice, and evaluation of the phenomenological method as a qualitative research procedure. *Journal of Phenomenological Psychology* 28, 235–260.

Halldorsdottir S. and Karlsdottir S. (1996) Empowerment or discouragement: women's experience of caring and uncaring encounters during childbirth. *Health Care Women International* 17, 361–379.

Hardin A.M. and Buckner E.B. (2004) Characteristics of a positive experience for women who have unmedicated childbirth. *Journal of Perinatal Education* 13, 10–16.

Heaton J. (2004) *Reworking Qualitative Data.* Sage Publications: London.

Heidegger M. (1998/1927) *Being and Time.* Blackwell: Oxford.

Hildingsson I., Waldenström U. and Rådestad I. (2003) Swedish women's interest in home birth and in-hospital birth centre care. *Birth* 30, 11–22.

Hildingsson I.M., Lindgren H.E., Haglund B. and Rådestad I.J. (2006) Characteristics of women giving birth at home in Sweden: a national register study. *Americacan Journal Obstetrics and Gynecology* 195, 1366–1372.

Hodnett E.D., Downe S., Edwards N. and Walsh D. (2005) *Home-like Versus Conventional Institutional Settings for Birth.* Cochrane Database of Systematic Reviews: London.

Hodnett E.D., Gates S., Hofmeyr G.J. and Sakala C. (2007) *Continuous Support for Women during Childbirth.* Cochrane Database of Systematic Reviews: London.

Hunter L.P. (2002) Being with woman: a guiding concept for the care of laboring women. *Journal of Obstetric, Gynecologic and Neonatal Nursing* 31, 650–657.

Husserl E. (1979) *The Crisis of European Sciences and Transcendental Phenomenology. An Introduction to Phenomenological Philosophy.* Northwestern University Press: Evanston.

Kennedy H.P. (1995) The essence of nurse-midwifery care. The woman's story. *Journal of Nurse-Midwifery* 40, 410–417.

Kennedy H.P., Shannon M.T., Chuahorm U.M. and Kravetz, K. (2004) The landscape of caring for women: A narrative study of midwifery practice. *Journal of Midwifery Women's Health* 49 (1), 14–23.

Kirkham M. (2003) Birth centre as an enabling culture. In: *Birth centres: A Social Model for Maternity Care* (ed. M. Kirkham), pp. 249–260. Books for Midwives: London.

Lahood G. (2007) Rumour of angels and heavenly midwives: Anthropology of transpersonal events and childbirth. *Women and Birth* 20, 3–10.

Larkin P., Begley C. and Devane D. (2009) Women's experiences of labour and birth: an evolutionary concept analysis. *Midwifery* 25, 49–59.

Lundgren I. (2002) Releasing and relieving encounters. Experiences of pregnancy and childbirth. (Doctoral dissertation). Uppsala University: Uppsala, Sweden.

Lundgren I. (2004) Releasing and relieving encounters: experiences of pregnancy and childbirth. *Scandinavian Journal of Caring Sciences* 18, 368–375.

Lundgren I. (2005) Swedish women's experience of childbirth 2 years after birth. *Midwifery* 21, 346–354.

Lundgren I. (2010) Women's experiences of giving birth and making decisions whether to give birth at home when professional care at home is not an option in public health care. *Sexual and Reproductive Healthcare* 1, 61–66.

Lundgren I., Karlsdottir S. and Bondas T. (2009) Long-term memories and experiences of childbirth in a Nordic context: a secondary analysis. *International Journal of Qualitative Studies on Health and Well-being* 4, 115–128.

Lynch E. (2007) Do-it-yourself delivery. *Nursing Standard* 22, 22–23.

Maslow A. (1979) *Religion, Values and Peak Experiences.* Viking: New York.

Merleau-Ponty M. (1995) *Phenomenology of Perception.* Routledge: London.

Milan M. (2003) Childbirth as healing: three women's experiences of independent midwife care. *Complementary Therapies in Nursing and Midwifery* 9, 160–166.

Nilsson C., Bondas T. and Lundgren I. (2010) Previous birth experience in women with intense fear of childbirth. *Journal of Obstetric, Gynecologic and Neonatal Nursing* 39 (3), 298–309.

Nolan M. (2008) Freebirthing: why on earth would women choose it? *The Practising Midwife* 11, 16–17.

Olafsdottir O.A. (2006) *An Icelandic Midwifery Saga – Coming to light: 'With woman' and Connective Ways of Knowing* (Unpublished PhD thesis). Thames Valley University: London.

Page L. (2003) One-to-one midwifery: Restoring the 'with woman' relationship in midwifery. *Journal of Midwifery and Women's Health* 48, 119–125.

Pairman S. (2006) Midwifery partnership working with women. In: *The New Midwifery: Science and Sensitivity in Practice* (eds L.A. Page and R. McCandlish), 73–97, Churchill Livingstone: Edinburgh.

Sawyer A. and Ayers S. (2009) Post-traumatic growth in women after childbirth. *Psychology and Health* 24, 457–471.

Simkin P. (1991) Just another day in a woman's life? Women's long-term perceptions of their first birth experience. Part I. *Birth* 18, 203–210.

Soet J., Brack G. and Dilorio C. (2003) Prevalence and predictors of women's experience of psychological trauma during childbirth. *Birth* 30, 36–46.

Stevens T. (2003) *Midwife to Mid Wife: A Study of Caseload Midwifery* (Doctoral dissertation). Thames Valley University: London.

Stockholms läns landsting (Stockholm county) (2002) Riktlinjer för ersättning från landstinget för hemförlossning (Guidelines for compensation for homebirth). Available online at www.sll.se/sll/templates/agendaitempage.aspx?id=14326.

Swedish Health Care Act (2003) *The Act Concerning the Ethical Review of Research Involving Humans: Vetting the Ethics of Research Involving Humans.* Retrieved October 10, 2009, from http://www.epn.se/start/startpage.aspx

Thomson G. and Downe S. (2008) Widening the trauma discourse: the link between child birth and experiences of abuse. *Journal of Psychosomatic Obstetrics and Gynecology* 29, 268–273.

Thorne S. (1994) Secondary analysis in qualitative research. In: *Critical Issues in Qualitative Research Methods* (ed. J.M. Morse), 263–279, Sage: Thousand Oaks.

Waldenström U., Hildingsson I., Ryding E.L. (2006) Antenatal *fear of childbirth* and its association with subsequent caesarean section and experience *of childbirth. International Journal of Obstetrics and Gynaecology* 113, 638–646.

8 'Abandonment of Being' in childbirth

Gill Thomson

Introduction

Childbirth is one of the most significant rites of passage in a woman's life and has long-term implications for maternal wellbeing. Over the last few centuries, childbirth in western society for most women has largely changed from a home-based experience to a hospital event. Over this period, an increasing number of women have been attended by formally qualified professionals. There has been a proliferation of commercially developed technical devices designed to aid or to speed up the labouring process. A range of sociological and anthropological authors have explored the rise in, and implications of, the use of modern technology in the childbirth arena. In this paper, I have drawn upon Heidegger's views of the dehumanizing implications of technology and 'machination' in modern society. Through re-analysis of an interpretive phenomenological research study into women's experiences of a traumatic birth, I offer a philosophically based discussion of how 'machination' has created an 'abandonment of Being' in childbirth.

Background

Since the introduction of the enlightenment sciences during the seventeenth century, a positivist epistemology has dominated scientific research (Ironside 2005). The basic premise of this approach is that there is a 'truth' which can be objectively measured through the deconstruction and statistical measurement of discrete variables. Positivism is also frequently argued to be the basis of modern obstetric practice (Martin 1987, Wertz and Wertz 1989, Davis-Floyd 1992). In this context it is elided with medicalization, and used with reference to an objective, delineated scientific approach in which a woman's body is subjected to increasingly sophisticated technologies, with little consideration of her expectations or experiences.

Anthropologist Emily Martin (1987) constructed the 'body as machine' metaphor to conceptualize the separation of body and mind in obstetric practice. The mechanical metaphor was created in seventeenth and eighteenth century French hospitals when the womb was deconstructed as a pump, and was subsequently re-conceptualized as part of a machine. This ideology was reinforced by the tools (forceps) which were developed to attend to the faulty machine (womb) (Martin 1987, p. 54). By replacing hands with tools, this served to reinforce women's alienation from their birth experience. Arney (1982) suggested that the medical professional project had to change the meaning of pregnancy and childbirth so that women would request specialized physician services. In this reading of events, childbirth was re-conceptualized from a normal physiological experience to an uncontrollable, potentially pathological process which required medical knowledge and expertise.

It has also been argued that the re-visioning of childbirth as a dangerous event also reinforced western modernist/consumerist society's fundamental belief about the superiority of technology over nature (Davis-Floyd 1992). This subsequently led to the development of increasingly more sophisticated technologies, with science used to cement pregnancy in a pathological realm (Arney 1982). These authors argue that the use of technology and expert opinion became integrated throughout a woman's pre-, intra- and post-partum period. The management of birth was deconstructed into a series of precise and effective manipulations and interventions designed to prevent and cure 'disease' (abnormality) (Wertz and Wertz 1989).

In this account of modernist childbirth, the extended control of obstetricians meant that all aspects of childbirth became subject to the 'medical gaze' (Foucault 2003). Within *The Birth of a Clinic*, Foucault (2003) refers to the creation of normalization within the medical profession. He highlights how the spirit of technology, through its rituals and techniques, has normalized the medical gaze to create a shared power base over individuals. The medical gaze therefore determined a particular version of reality for all who operated within it. Arney (1982), in adopting a Foucauldian perspective argued that the surveillance and monitoring equipment in maternity practice created the 'new order of social control' (p. 91). This social control is considered to have blurred the boundaries in defining normal and abnormal birth as babies, women and obstetricians became subject to the monitoring regimes.

These sociological and anthropological authors offer interesting and illuminating insights into how technological progress has influenced maternity services. However, it is significant to reflect that Heidegger was one of the early thinkers to identify the negative implications of technology (Todres *et al.* 2007) in western society. Heidegger considered that technological progress had culminated in the dominance of technological and calculable ways of thinking and handling objects, a state he refers to as 'machination' (Heidegger 1977). Through machination all entities become raw materials for quantitative measurement, calculation and control:

Machination is not just a human behaviour, the act of manipulation; it is a revelation of beings as a whole as exploitable and manipulable objects.

(Polt 2003, p. 142)

Heidegger's concern was not towards an instrumental view of technology as tools and products to be used, but rather the 'essence' of technology. From a purely instrumental perspective, technology is viewed as something that can be mastered. The 'essence' of technology relates to the means through which concealed energy from nature is reduced into a 'standing reserve' (a resource that can be manipulated or controlled) (Carnevale 2005). Heidegger refers to this process as 'enframing': a process through which nature is contained by humans solely to serve the instrumental ends of humans (Heidegger 1977). His apprehension related to how the 'essence' of technology, the cause and effect nature of enframing, disintegrated and concealed the essence of 'truth' of human existence (Carnevale 2005):

Enframing challenges forth into the frenzied-ness of ordering that blocks every view into the coming-to-pass of revealing and so radically endangers the relation to the essence of truth.

(Heidegger 1977, p. 33)

According to Heidegger, machination has become the exclusive view through which the world and the 'truth' of entities are 'unconcealed' (as objective statements of facts) whilst subsequently concealing other ways of understanding the world, such as nature, in its entirety. He did not consider technological progress to be detrimental *per se*, just that in constantly choosing technology over other modes of being, we sacrificed other ways of 'Being-in-the-world':

Modern technology is too a means to an end. That is why the instrumental conception of technology conditions every attempt to bring man into the right relation to technology. Everything depends on our manipulating technology in the proper manner as a means.

(Heidegger 1977, p. 5)

Through our lack of questioning regarding our relationship to technology, Heidegger believed that technical ways of being were relentlessly overtaking humanity, creating technical nihilism through its ability to alter our existence. This nature–scientific mode of understanding has subsequently led to an ever-increasing abandonment of Being or 'forgotten-ness' of human existence (which Heidegger referred to as the 'darkening of the world'). He described three principal concealments of 'machination': 'calculation', 'acceleration' and the 'outbreak of massiveness' (Heidegger 1976, p. 121).

In the findings section below, these underpinning concepts are described and discussed in relation to how an epoch of machination has led to an abandonment of Being in childbirth.

Methodology

Theoretical perspective

The aim of my research was to explore the lived experiences of women who had experienced a self-defined traumatic birth followed by a positive experience of childbirth. I chose an interpretive phenomenological approach based on the philosophical works of Martin Heidegger and Hans-Georg Gadamer as my theoretical perspective. This approach was adopted as Heidegger's phenomenological analysis offers a reflective and open approach to explore and interpret phenomenon. Furthermore, Heidegger has provided meaningful insights into how our 'Dasein' interprets our ontological and ontic lifeworld through Being-in-the-world (also discussed in Chapters 3 and 12).

Martin Heidegger's life-long phenomenological quest was to answer the question of the meaning of 'Being'. Heidegger distinguished between 'Being' as the primordial (ontological) meaningful structure of existence and 'being' which refers to the 'ontic' concrete, factual representations of entities. Heidegger (1962) argued that to understand Being one must first understand the human kind of being referred to as 'Dasein'. Dasein is the kind of being who asks the question of Being (Heidegger 1962). The term 'Dasein' is literally translated as 'being-there'. According to Heidegger, before anything else, we exist; we are 'there' in the world. To stress the importance of this concept, Heidegger referred to Dasein's activity of existence as Being-in-the-world. Our 'there' is so essential that there is no existing, no 'being-there' without a world in which to exist.

The findings of this study uncovered how women experienced and internalized trauma, and how they were moved from a state of despair and grief to the joy and elation of a subsequent positive birth experience (refer to Thomson and Downe 2008, Thomson and Downe 2010, Thomson 2010). In this chapter I have re-analysed the women's traumatic birth narratives drawing on Heidegger's conception of 'machination' to discuss how technological progress has led to an abandonment of Being in childbirth.

Participants

A purposive sampling method recruited 14 women aged between 35 to 40 years over two recruitment phases. Phase-one participants had already experienced both a self-defined traumatic and positive birth ($n = 10$). Two of the women did not specifically match the recruitment profile. One woman had only one traumatic birth. The other woman had two positive births followed by a traumatic birth. These women were included to consider differences between women who end their childbearing on trauma or joy. In phase two, pregnant women who had previously experienced a traumatic birth ($n = 4$) were recruited. All women were recruited through the consultant midwife based at one maternity unit in England.

All women gave birth to healthy full-term babies. The traumatic birth experiences involved forceps ($n = 5$), caesareans ($n = 5$) and uncomplicated vaginal deliveries ($n = 4$). With regard to positive birth experiences, nine were uncomplicated vaginal deliveries, four were caesarean sections ($n = 4$, two elective and two unplanned), and one was a forceps delivery. These women were interviewed some 18 months to 19 years following their traumatic births.

Procedure

Participants were invited to participate in the study by the consultant midwife and provided with an information sheet and reply slip. Once the completed reply slip was received, an interview was organized.

Data collection

Phase-one participants ($n = 10$) were engaged in two in-depth interviews (data collection and interpretation interview). Phase-two participants ($n = 4$) were engaged in three interviews: two data collection interviews (one at 36 weeks gestation and one at three months postnatally) and one interpretation interview. All interviews were undertaken during August 2005 to November 2006. Interviews were held at the participant's home ($n = 27$), my home ($n = 2$) or the woman's place of work ($n = 3$).

At the data collection interviews, women were presented with a broad, open-ended question: 'Please can you tell me about your childbirth experience(s), and your feelings and perceptions towards this/these experiences?' After the woman had finished reciting her story, numerous open prompt questions were posed to explore the key issues disclosed. After each interview I recorded my thoughts and feelings in a field notes journal.

Following initial data analysis, all the women were engaged in an 'interpretation interview'. During this interview women were presented with the thematic areas arising from the initial data collection phase, followed by in-depth exploration and discussion of these issues. This was a highly useful and insightful exercise as it enabled a much richer exploration of meanings.

All interviews were audio-taped and transcribed in full.

Ethical considerations

Ethics approval was obtained through the local NHS Research Ethics Committee (REC), and the sponsoring University Ethics Committee. All participants were informed about the voluntary nature of participation. The information collected was treated as strictly confidential, and pseudonyms used within public accounts. Protocols were in place to refer the women to appropriate personnel within or outside of the Trust (should anxiety/distress be experienced).

An unexpected ethical issue emerged concerning child protection, which subsequently led to the initiation of safeguarding procedures (for personal reflections on this experience refer to Anon 2006). Following this encounter, I revised my paperwork to stipulate that further actions would be taken should 'issues of concern' be disclosed. The project was reassessed and approval granted by REC.

Data analysis

In this section I outline an overview of the analytical stages I adopted for this research. Rather than a rule-governed sequential logic, they offer a descriptive process to represent the circular and reflexive nature of an interpretive phenomenological enquiry.

Explication of pre-understandings

Heidegger (1962) and Gadamer (2004) conceived that the only way human beings are able to interpret and comprehend their lifeworld is through their primordial pre-understandings ('horizon'). Furthermore, these presuppositions are not rigid entities, but they are mediated and developed through the confrontation of new meanings. At the start of the research my pre-understandings of childbirth on a personal, theoretical and conceptual basis were recorded in a reflexive journal. Alterations to these a priori assumptions were documented on an ongoing basis to maintain an open and reflective attitude.

Submersion within phenomena

Gadamer (2004) believed that the acquisition of knowledge and interpretation requires immersion within the subject matter. My methods of submersion included my personal experiences, in-depth interviews with participants, experiential descriptions within the literature as well as other informants (secondary sources), key academic literature and artistic depictions.

Fusion of horizons (exposition of themes)

Understanding is achieved through co-constructed agreements (Gadamer 2004). A 'fusion of horizons' occurs between the interpreter and what is interpreted. Furthermore, the aim of an interpretive phenomenological enquiry is to identify resonant themes that create a pattern of understanding (Diekelmann and Magnussen-Ironside 1998). In my study, analysis involved successive listening and reading of the narratives. A mapping framework was created to document the 'naïve' concepts that emerged. All scripts were then assessed against the framework, with modifications made as appropriate. Every single sentence and section of each text was then assessed to expose meanings of the phenomena. This stage of analysis was highly iterative, moving from basic concepts and themes to a deeper cyclical action generating firmer meanings and interpretations.

Rich descriptions of phenomenon

The last stage was the creation of a detailed and comprehensive understanding of the phenomenon. Paradigm cases, exemplars and passages representative of the shared understandings were chosen to illuminate and frame the themes constructed. Finally, the interpretations were interwoven with existing research and other relevant explanatory literature to enhance the meanings generated.

Findings and discussion

In this chapter, I have re-analysed women's experiences of their self-defined traumatic births. Details of the themes and patterns of understanding generated through this work have been published elsewhere (Thomson and Downe 2008, Thomson 2010, Thomson and Downe 2010). For this analysis, I have used Heideggerian insights to illuminate how technological progress and the epoch of 'machination' has led to an abandonment of Being in childbirth.

A number of the women in this study experienced complications during their traumatic birth (such as pre-eclampsia, *Streptococcus B* and complications with the foetal presentation). In the following interpretations I do not wish to convey that technology was unnecessary; rather in line with Heidegger's thoughts, technology was problematic due to *how* it was used:

> [it is] the human distress caused by the technological understanding of Being, rather than the destruction caused by specific technologies.
>
> (Dreyfus 1993, p. 305)

Heidegger considered that there were three underpinning influences of machination which have to led an abandonment of Being. These relate to the outbreak of massiveness, calculation and acceleration. In the findings I have used these concepts as the basis of the interpretations. Each interpretive theme provides a brief description of the Heideggerian concept together with a discussion of how these influences are evident during a traumatic birth, contextualized by quotes from the women's narratives. These interpretations offer insights into how technologically imbued procedures and practices have standardized, depersonalized and objectified women's bodies; with minimal consideration of the emotional and value-laden nature of childbirth and motherhood.

In the final thematic area, I offer a more generalized discussion of how technological progress (and associated ordering, manipulation and control of women's bodies) has led to an abandonment of Being during childbirth. Within this exposition, I have also drawn upon a number of Heidegger's ontological insights to consider the socio-cultural context in which an epoch of machination has been created within maternity care.

Outbreak of massiveness

Outbreak of massiveness relates to how technology has rendered 'beings' to be perceived as prescribed, lineated and homogenous resources:

> what is common to the many and to all
>
> (Heidegger 1976, p. 79)

Through 'enframing', 'beings' (including the human 'being') are turned over into a standing-reserve of resources which is streamlined and uniformly equated with every other 'being' through specific rules and procedures. In maternity care the enframing of women's bodies occurs through clinical checks, scans, vaginal examinations and electrocardiographs, which serve to expose women's bodies as a standardized and homogenous resource. Numerous clinical standards, procedures and protocols have also been established to dictate 'normality' and govern how 'correct' childbirth should be managed. These rules and procedures thereby determine how the 'resources' (women's bodies) should be controlled based on objective 'truths':

> the demand for rules is a symptom of the technological approach to the world, an approach that tries to manage and control the behaviour of all entities, including human beings.
>
> (Polt 2003, p. 169)

On one hand these guidelines offer parameters of safety and care. From a counter perspective they have created prototypes of responses through which individual and unique patterns are discarded. In this study, some women spoke of their inherent knowledge being subjugated when their bodies failed to meet objectively determined standards of progress:

> I had it in my head that I was soft because they kept sending me home, "oh you're not in established labour, you're only 1 cm dilated". I'm thinking god, get a grip, saying to my mum I don't know how I'm going to cope when I'm in labour.
>
> (Jules)

Within a traumatic birth, the supra-ordination of technology over women's bodies was evident with professionals *'rushing in and out'* to attend to the machines: often with minimal dialogue, explanation or care provided to women:

> they were just looking at your cervix or your blood pressure, I never felt that they understood my situation or were even sort of very interested in it.
>
> (Jackie)

The women's bodies were often 'exposed' (naked) and rendered passive and compliant (through machines, procedures and medication) to the control and manipulation of technology. This was explicitly described by Holly:

> they [health professionals] just like told me how I was feeling – "oh no this is, this is what you need, this is what you'll be feeling right now"…. and it was like telling me what I should be doing, how I should be feeling, and I wanted to move, because, I was in agony just being led on the bed all the time, I was strapped to these monitors, and "oh no, no, you've got to lie on that bed you've got to, you've got to stay on that bed, you can't move anywhere" and ….they restricted me in every way, shape or form.
>
> (Holly)

These insights resonate with Heidegger's criticisms of technology in terms of how it represented a 'will to will'. For a number of the women in my study these procedures often offered no purpose apart from 'self-assertion and sheer power' (Polt 2003, p. 173). Women's Dasein, their values, feelings and concerns often went unvalued and unrecognized. The alienation and subjugation of their identity rendered them as a 'faceless', 'empty body':

> to talk to you like you're a person, not a baby incubator, just a lump of meat.
>
> (Kate)

According to Heidegger, the outbreak of massiveness is where quantifiable 'truths' are utilized as the prototype of standards and responses which can manipulate and dominate the standing reserves. This is achieved through the processes of calculation and acceleration.

Calculation

Heidegger's concept of calculation refers to calculable objective measurements of progress and success:

> All 'beings' are determined and organised by guiding principles and rules; everything is regulated through calculation.
>
> (Vallega-Neu 2003, p. 59)

During childbirth enframing involved the calculation and measurement of women's bodily responses. Manufactured clock time is also utilized to calculate the boundaries of when women can give birth (Downe and Dykes 2009). Protocols dictate that childbirth should occur within a specific time period following rupture of the membranes and for cervical dilatation to progress at approximately 1 cm an hour. In my study, a number of the women spoke of running '*out of time*' due to these obligatory standards of normality:

> I knew I was going to have a caesarean after 24 hours.
>
> (Jill)

Linear time was also utilized to determine when medication should be provided irrespective of the woman's physiological pain:

> I was just lying down and the pain was getting worse, and I was being told that I couldn't have anything until I was over 1.5 cms dilated. One of the doctors or midwives said "well this could go on for 72 hours you could be in labour at this stage for hours, so you can't have anything"
>
> (Jackie)

Problems were often experienced in how women's progress was calculated, and how this information was utilized to undermine the labouring woman. For instance, women spoke of how their assenting bodies would endure '*intrusive*' vaginal examinations (often performed by numerous professionals) only to have their bodily responses negated:

> it was a case of every three hours somebody coming in the room with rubber gloves on and shove their hand up and say you're still 4 cms.
>
> (Lesley)

Health professionals frequently utilized negative terminology to convey the women's lack of measurable progress during labour. Phrases such as 'oh you're only', 'you're not much further' and 'this baby's never going to be born' were regular occurrences within the traumatic birth narratives:

> Because I think the thing that gets you through the pain is thinking that it's doing good and your cervix is opening and the baby's going to be born. So then when somebody comes in after all that time and pain and says "oh no it's not, it's not done anything", you just think well what was the point in that.
>
> (Janet)

Following this interaction Janet asked for a caesarean section to be performed.

Heidegger refers to language as 'the house of Being' (Polt 2003, p. 175). It is the fundamental means through which we come to comprehend and understand our Being-in-the-world:

> Language is the medium in which Being takes hold of us, appropriates us, and allows us and all beings to come into our own.
>
> (Polt 2003, p. 178)

In these narratives, the language served to highlight the defective nature of the woman's body and it introduced risk and fear into their birth experience. The power of language coupled with the rules of calculation undermined women's self-capabilities and beliefs as they surrendered their bodies to technological control.

Acceleration

Acceleration refers to the (artificial) speeding up of processes to achieve the desired outcomes. In this study, almost all had experienced augmentation of their labour. The endless optimization imperative of enframing meant that when abnormality was unconcealed, professionals intervened to control and speed up the women's physiological responses. However, this was often performed without the women's informed consent:

> what he [doctor] actually did was sweep my membranes, but never told me what he was going to do, I had no idea what he was going to do and it was really really painful and I nearly like broke X's [husband] fingers. He didn't ask me if he could do it, he didn't explain what he was doing and that stayed with me ever since really, it felt very intrusive and even abusive.
>
> (Jules)

Acceleration is referred to as 'and not-being-able-to-bear the stillness of hidden growth' (Heidegger 1976, p. 84). The process of acceleration meant that the hidden growth in women's bodies was often disregarded. As technology is unable to 'unconceal' or predict natural physiological progress, professionals intervened and speeded-up the birth in line with its totalizing all-engulfing standards.

For a number of these women, the acceleration of their contractions rendered them vulnerable and increasingly dependent on professional care due to an inability to control their bodily responses. The violence and force in which these procedures were applied often created a scenario of 'torture' and 'abuse' (Thomson and Downe 2008):

> all three [Janet, her husband and her mother] of us have said it was like being tortured because I was led on the bed screaming, with the monitors on... begging, really really begging for it [Syntocin drip] to be turned off, and she [midwife] were just turning it up all the time.
>
> (Janet)

Augmentation was commonly associated with the administration of pain relief and often culminated in operative and medical deliveries. Women's choices and values were disregarded as their bodies were attended to with increasing speed and urgency. This was described by Diane:

> she broke my waters and found that there was meconium in the waters and said that they needed to do an induction and put me on the drip, and I sort of questioned it at the time and I started to feel a bit uneasy but I had to go with it because they said that needed to get me going because things weren't happening and my blood pressure was too high. I didn't want all the drugs and everything, but, when you're faced with something, you've never been through before, you don't know medically how things are going to affect you, I had to go with what they were saying....people were telling me what needed to happen to me and I couldn't let my body take the control it needed to take to give birth to her, because outsiders were coming in taking that away.
>
> (Diane)

Similar to Heidegger's conceptions of technology, in maternity care acceleration was utilized 'to drive the maximum yield at the minimum expense' (Heidegger 1977, p. 15) for women's Dasein.

Abandonment of Being

According to Heidegger, machination turns 'Being' into 'present-at-hand' beings (Heidegger 1977). This is when the perceiver is concerned with the bare facts and concepts that are presented, and there is no concern for the history, value or usefulness of the being. In a traumatic birth, enframing rendered women's bodies as re-presentable and calculable 'present-at-hand' objects. Women's abandonment of Being was illuminated by how they did not feel they had given birth to their infant (Thomson and Downe 2008, Thomson and Downe 2010). Childbirth was '*done to them*' and '*for them*':

> This birth experience was taken from me and somebody else delivered me, delivered my baby.
>
> (Ann)

The essence of technology thereby concealed the essence of Being a mother.

In order to understand how machination has created a 'forgottenness of Being' it is useful to consider Heidegger's concepts of 'thrownness', 'Being-with' and 'inauthenticity'. Whilst it is appreciated that Heidegger describes these as higher-order concepts which are subjectively determined, they do provide the means to illuminate the socio-cultural context in which an epoch of machination can exist in maternity services. These concepts are now outlined, followed by a description of their relevance to maternity care. Furthermore, the use of the women's quotes in this section have been utilized to highlight the specific points being considered; rather than as a definitive interpretation of Heidegger's philosophy.

As discussed by Healy in Chapter 12, 'thrownness' relates to how we are 'thrown' into a world of understanding (our 'tradition'). It is our heritage of enculturation into a shared community at a specific historical period. It provides the primordial basis through which we are able to engage with and make meaning of our lifeworld (Heidegger 1962). Heidegger also considered that as human beings, we are always 'Being-with' others, the 'they' ['das Man'] (Heidegger 1962). Being-in-the-world is a 'Being-with'. As we live in a world shared with 'the-they', self-understanding occurs in relation to how others affect our notion of self (Smythe 2002, p. 173).

Our thrownness provides a number of options. Heidegger considered it was through 'concern' that we decide which decisions to make. On an individual level we are concerned about our own Being and what is 'at stake' for us (Polt 2003). Therefore, whilst we live out our existence through concern, Heidegger believed that we may exist within one of two modes; an authentic or inauthentic existence. An authentic existence is whereby we do not fatefully accept what is handed down to us but seek our 'own-most potential to Being' (Heidegger 1962). An inauthentic existence is whereby we operate in the everyday of existence as 'the-they'. For Heidegger, one of the problems of Being-with is when we come to exist only in reference to others (also refer to Chapter 12). We become lost in an anonymous, formless and inauthentic 'they-ness'. Heidegger describes this inauthentic state as 'fallenness'. Fallenness is also perceived to be the fundamental basis of our thrownness; the primordial nature of our Being-in-the-world (Heidegger 1962):

Dasein's falling into the 'they' and the 'world' of its concerns, is that we have called a 'fleeing' in the face of itself.

(Heidegger 1962, p. 230)

In consideration of these concepts with the women's narratives, their thrownness provided them with pre-suppositions about childbirth. In modern society, women go into hospitals to have their babies and health professionals facilitate childbirth. A few of the women had expectations of what they would achieve during their birth, whereas others held a '*wait and see*' attitude:

> I had this plan of I'll take it all as it comes I've no idea what to expect and I'll go off her (midwife) advice sort of thing, so I didn't have really a birth plan as such, I just said whatever I feel I'll need I'll have.
>
> (Lesley)

However, all the women held uncomplicated faith towards the professionals who would direct their care:

> I can remember my birth plan in what I would have like to have happened, but I was very open and wanted to be guided by their expertise. They are the experts, they do this day in day out, if they say I need such and such a thing, I need it.
>
> (Jules)

These insights reflect the fallenness of inauthenticity. The inherent suggestion within the narratives was that health professionals held expert status over childbirth, and they were willing to hand over responsibility to their caregivers. They also viewed health professionals as the authoritative 'they' who would facilitate an authentic birth outcome. However, the reality of a traumatic birth shattered these pre-judgements. Heidegger considered that it is profound moments when we can become alienated from our lifeworld, and 'fall' into decline. Through the disregard of their Dasein, women became 'not themselves' and surrendered their existence to the 'they-ness'. The risks exposed through enframing ensured the women's inauthentic compliance. It enabled health professionals to exert power over labouring women, irrespective of whether the perceived risk was felt justified:

> I had to go with what they were saying, we both questioned it we tried to question it but at the end of the day we didn't want X [daughter] at risk, even though all the way through it X's [daughter] little heart was ticketty-booing along, she wasn't distressed at all.
>
> (Diane)

Similar to Heidegger's conception of machination women experienced power and violence through 'impotent attempts to change entities without deeper insights or ontological attunement' (Dallmayr 2004, p. 109).

The paucity of information about why procedures were being performed and disregard of women's concerns also reflect Heidegger's characterization of fallenness as achieved through 'idle talk' and 'ambiguity' (Heidegger 1962):

> I put complete trust in the people that were looking after me, and I never doubted them, I never questioned them, I expected them to do their job and do it well. I did that to such an extent that I didn't reason and think well for God's sake this is not right, this is not reasonable, this level of pain for this long, letting someone go for a week without sleep....but I trusted them.
>
> (Jules)

Inauthentic Being-with was evident through the quality of relationships and connections forged between women and professionals. Women often described their caregivers as 'cold', 'harsh' 'uncaring' and 'clinical'. It represented care that was focused on instrumental rather than emotional based support (Thomson and Downe 2008). Reciprocal mistrust was also evident in the narratives. Women did not trust the care they received as the professionals mistrusted their bodies:

> It's just my overall impression that the midwives really didn't share my view that I could do it on my own, I think they were too keen to engage in interventions and not trying to get this baby out any other way than with a great big pair of scissors. I don't think enough effort was made by the midwives to let my body do the work, I think they wanted to do the work, it's their job.
>
> (Ann)

During their traumatic birth, women were often attended by numerous caregivers; however, this was not mentioned as often as the quality of care that left them feeling dissatisfied and '*betrayed*'.

Heidegger perceived that it is only in 'absence' are we truly aware of 'presence'. The absence of the women's expectations of childbirth and motherhood was painfully experienced in the postnatal period:

> [I was] just left alone just wondering what'd gone wrong, what had happened, why the birth turned out as it had – it was a very very sad time really when it should have been a happy experience, and I will never ever get over the fact that it was...[starts to cry]
>
> (Hannah)

Professionals also appeared to operate within a state of inauthenticity as they enforced the clinical standards and rules of their professional and cultural (hospital) existence. Heidegger conceived that an inauthentic Being creates a passive self who is disburdened of moral autonomy and responsibility. This perspective provides an appreciation of how professionals could dogmatically enforce procedures amid the screams, concerns and questions of labouring women.

Heidegger believes that technological understanding has transformed our relationships to others. The problem is that these transformations go unrecognized as the pervasiveness of machination has rendered them invisible. It is important to reflect that I do not suggest that compliance with rules and procedures is always inauthentic. Rather, the women's insights suggest that it was how technological practices and procedures were enforced without holistic consideration of the women's Dasein that rendered these practices to be inauthentic. In my study, the health professionals appeared to operate in they-ness, with minimal questioning or regard for the women's Being:

> I think because they [health professionals] deal with it all the time so I think they must get used to people screaming and writhing around in agony and it doesn't affect them.
>
> (Jackie)

Health professionals therefore appeared to have become part of the standing-reserves utilized as implements to manipulate the resources (women's bodies). As the staff became inauthentically absorbed in technological processes and linear clock-based time, their own Dasein became abandoned and depersonalized:

> It's more a case of books and protocol and they're looking at this case and they're saying well this should happen now rather than looking at an individual case.....it's all very proceduralized.
>
> (Janet)

Inauthentic existence exists in a state of fear. Fear is always 'fear of something and for the sake of something' (Heidegger 1962, p. 179). Fear is a state through which rational thought becomes compromised and one clings to safety and defensiveness. During a traumatic birth fear was instilled through risks, pathological pain, clinical interventions, lack of control and a lack of care. Over half the women felt at some point that they were going to die, with two women welcoming death as an end to their torment (Thomson and Downe 2008). Heidegger considered that we are always 'Being-towards-death' and an acceptance of our finitude can project us into an authentic existence. In these women's stories, it was fear that forced them to face their finitude creating deeply psychic disturbances:

I think when you think you're going to die and really believe that you're facing your own death I don't think your life is ever the same again and I think in stressful situations I analyse things a lot more, I think I'm more aware of death and illness and hospitals – definitely more frightened of them.

(Jules)

Fear was also evident in women's unwillingness to complain in case of potential retribution on their subsequent care, reflecting the power imbalance in these technologically enforced relationships:

It's like how you can you complain when you have no power...they [professionals] have all the power.

(Kate)

The inherent notion of risk and abnormality within childbirth has been associated with the litigation culture of modern society. Threats of litigation are perceived to encourage the use of medical technology to ensure control, predictability and safety (Walsh *et al.* 2004). Fear of safety and litigation appeared to create the fallenness of inauthenticity experienced during a traumatic birth. Women and professionals become deprived of their own accountability as technological-based procedures identify and manage potential risks on present-at-hand bodies.

Methodological challenges

The strengths of an interpretive phenomenological approach are that it offers rich and meaningful insights into lived experiences of phenomenon. Heideggerian phenomenological analysis offers the basis for an open, circular and reflexive attitude to interpretations and insightful meanings of our Being-in-the-world.

As outlined within all the chapters in this book, phenomenological interpretations are never finite and unending. As we comprehend something anew, this provides us with a new horizon of understanding. Whilst interpretive phenomenology makes explicit that it is our pre-suppositions and pre-judgements that renders the world meaningful, it is important that these do not mask, or make incomplete, judgements about what is being perceived. In my research, I 'laid-bare' my prejudices within a reflexive diary, which subsequently became subject to ongoing reflections as data collection and interpretations progressed. I re-visited the participants, shared my insights with my supervision team and talked to professional and lay service user groups about my insights. I can appreciate how my personal experience of a medicalized birth became an integral feature of these interpretations; however, with an open attitude and iterative, inquisitive approach, they can offer one interpretation, from a specific group of women, at a specific historical moment.

Implications

These insights reflect how the technological progress of the maternity care can lead to a withdrawal or 'forgottenness of Being' (Heidegger 1977). The dominance of technological and calculable ways of thinking have obscured and 'concealed' even the possibility of any question about the essence and nature of Being (childbirth) itself.

Heidegger's view was not to destroy the machines. Rather he called for technical devises to be used as they ought to be used and in ways in which they do not affect 'our inner and real core' (Polt 2003, p. 174). In maternity care, there is a necessity for technology (equipment, rules and procedures) to be used sensitively and in harmony with women's bodies. Technology needs to be explained, accepted and consented to by women. There is a need for 'letting-be' (Heidegger 1976) to allow 'truth' to be unconcealed in women's natural physiological responses; rather than 'leaping-in' to respond to the hegemony of 'truth as correctness':

> ...letting-be involves waiting, listening, responding – attentively receiving what is given to us.
>
> (Polt 2003, p. 173)

The benefits of 'being with' women through the provision of sensitive and individualized care has been well reported within the maternity literature (refer to Hunter (2002), Kennedy *et al.* (2004), Edwards (2005)). From a Heideggerian perspective it urges for Being-with to be authentically provided. Authentic existence occurs when we realize who we are, we take 'responsibility' for our actions and can grasp that each human being is a distinctive Being. In maternity care, health professionals need to value the significance of childbirth and Be-with a woman so that their Dasein is perceived in its entirety; as a mother with individually determined responses, values and beliefs.

Conclusion

Heidegger's state of machination is evident within women's traumatic birth narratives. Women are rendered as a technological Dasein, a present-at-hand object that is available for exploitation and manipulation, with technologically-imbued processes (as well as professionals) becoming the manipulator and exploiter of the object. Through the underpinning influences of the outbreak of massiveness, calculation and acceleration women's bodies were objectively subjected to ever-increasing efficiency and control. Through fear, women and health professionals operated in an inauthentic mode of existence. This created an absence and concealment of the essential meanings of childbirth. Machination's all-engulfing framework of conceptualization and calculation ultimately led to women's as well as health professionals' abandonment of Being.

Heidegger calls for a 'new beginning' (Heidegger 1977). He did not want technology destroyed; rather he considers that we need to achieve a balance that keeps technology in its place:

To use machines as they work with nature, instead of assaulting it.

(Polt 2003, p. 174)

In maternity care, this suggests a need to balance technology with an authentic Being-with. This can free women and health professionals to experience what has been forgotten – the 'truth of Being' in childbirth.

References

Anon (2006) Unexpected ethical issues emerging from research: a case in point. *British Journal of Midwifery* 14 (4), 150.

Arney, W.R. (1982) *Power and the Profession of Obstetrics.* The University of Chicago Press: London.

Carnevale, F.A. (2005) The palliation of dying: a Heideggerian analysis of the 'technologization' of death. *The Indo-Pacific Journal of Phenomenology* 5(1). [online]. Available from: http://www.ipjp.org/april2005/carnevale_5e1.pdf [Accessed 20 May, 2007].

Dallmayr, F. (2004) The underside of modernity: Adorno, Heidegger and Dussel. *Consellations* 11(1), 102–120.

Davis-Floyd, R. (1992) *Birth as an American Rite of Passage.* University of California Press: Berkeley.

Diekelmann, N.L. and Ironside, P.M. (1998) Preserving writing in doctoral education: Exploring the concernful practices of schooling learning teaching. *Journal of Advanced Nursing*, 28(6), 1347–1355.

Downe, S. and Dykes, F. (2009) Counting Time in Pregnancy and Labour. In *Childbirth, Midwifery and Concepts of Time* (ed. C. McCourt). Berghaun Books: London.

Dreyfus, R. (1993) 'Heidegger on the connection between nililism, art, technology and politics'. In *The Cambridge Companion to Heidegger* (ed. C. Guigon). Cambridge University Press: Cambridge.

Edwards, N.P. (2005) *Birthing Autonomy: Women's Experiences of Planning Home Births.* Routledge Press: London.

Foucault, M. (2003) *The Birth of a Clinic.* Routledge Press: London.

Gadamer, H.G. (2004) *Truth and Method.* Continuum Press: London.

Heidegger, M. (1962) *Being and Time.* Harper & Row Publishers: New York.

Heidegger, M. (1976) *Contributions to Philosophy (From Enowning)* (trans. Parvis, E. and Kenneth, M.). Indiana University Press: Bloomington.

Heidegger, M. (1977) *The Question Concerning Technology and Other Essays.* Harper & Row: New York.

Hunter, L.P. (2002) Being with woman: A guiding concept for the care of laboring women'. *Journal of Obstetric, Gynecologic and Neonatal Nursing* 31(6), 650–657.

Ironside, P. (2005) *Beyond Method: Philosophical Conversations in Healthcare Research and Scholarship. Volume 4 Interpretive Studies in Healthcare and the Human Sciences,* ix–xix. University of Wisconsin Press: Wisconsin.

Kennedy, H.P., Shannon, M.T., Chuahorn, U. and Kravetz, M.K. (2004) The landscape of caring for women: A narrative study of midwifery practice. *American College of Nurse-Midwives* 49 (1), 14–23.

Martin, E. (1987) *The Woman in the Body: A Cultural Analysis of Reproduction.* Beacon Press: Boston.

Polt, R. (2003) *Heidegger: an Introduction.* Routledge Press: Oxon.

Smythe, E. (2002) The violence of the everyday in healthcare. In *First, Do No Harm: Power Oppression and Violence in Healthcare. Volume 1. Interpretive Studies in Healthcare and the Human Sciences* (ed. N. Diekelmann), 163–203. University of Wisconsin Press: Wisconsin.

Thomson, G. (2010) Birth as a Peak Experience. In *Intrapartum Care (Essential Midwifery Practice)* (eds D. Walsh and S. Downe). Wiley Blackwell Publishers: London.

Thomson, G. and Downe, S. (2008) Widening the trauma discourse: the link between childbirth and experiences of abuse. *Journal of Psychosomatic Obstetrics and Gynaecology* 29(4), 268–273.

Thomson, G. and Downe, S. (2010) Changing the future to change the past: women's experiences of a positive birth following a traumatic birth experience. *Journal of Reproductive and Infant Psychology* 28(1), 102–112.

Todres, L., Galvin, K. and Dahlberg, K. (2007) Lifeworld-led healthcare: revisiting a humanising philosophy that integrates emerging trends. *Medicine, Healthcare and Philosophy* 10, 53–63.

Vallega-Neu, D. (2003) *Heidegger's Contributions to Philosophy: An Introduction.* Indiana University Press: Bloomington.

Walsh, D., El-Nemer, A. and Downe, S. (2004) Risk, safety and the study of physiological birth. In *Normal Childbirth Evidence and Debate* (ed. S. Downe), 103–120. Churchill-Livingstone: China.

Wertz, R.C. and Wertz, D.C. (1989) *Lying-In: A History of Childbirth in America.* Yale University Press: New Haven, CT.

9 Parents' participation in the care of their child in neonatal intensive care

Marie Berg and Helena Wigert

Introduction

When people think about becoming a parent, they usually see it as a natural part of life, and they believe that the child will be born healthy. However, due to premature birth and illnesses some newborns require care in a neonatal intensive care unit (NICU). In this chapter we will present an interpretative synthesis of three lifeworld phenomenological studies related to parents' participation in the NICU care of their child.

Background

Becoming a mother and father involves a transition that includes several overwhelming feelings. The importance of an early, close mother–child relationship has been identified as central for the development of the child (Bowlby 1969, Ainsworth 1973, Klaus and Kennell 1982, Adshead and Bluglass 2005, Kennell and McGrath 2005). International policy documents state that all children regardless of age are entitled to have their parents with them throughout their stay in hospital (UNICEF 1989, NOBAB 1992). When a newborn child needs care at a NICU the essential relationship between the newborn and the parents is fragile. The parents are concerned about losing the child as well as the damaging effects of treatments or investigations (Franck and Spencer 2003, Heerman *et al.* 2005). They have not yet established a relationship with their child, and it has been reported that the way in which health care professionals treat them is significant in helping them to build this relationship (Cescutti-Butler and Galvin 2003).

According to the literature, health care professionals (HCPs) should invite parents to be partners in the care of the infant (Heerman *et al.* 2005, Griffin and Abraham 2006). Ideally, parents and HCPs should work in a mutual interaction to provide care for a child who needs to be in an NICU. According to the Swedish Children and Parents Code, parents are responsible for their child's wellbeing, and they have a right and duty to decide on issues concerning their child when cared for in hospital (Föräldrabalken 1949:381). In order to assume this responsibility, parents must be given the opportunity to be present and take part in their child's care. Parents on a NICU in Sweden are welcome to stay with and participate in the care of their child at all times. However, in other countries this practice is not always possible.

For decades as a paediatric nurse, the author (HW) has cared for new-born children and engaged and interacted with parents. As a nurse and a midwife the author (MB) has performed care for mothers during their postnatal hospital stay while their newborn was being cared for at a NICU. A common research interest between the authors of this chapter was mothers' experiences of separation from their infants in a NICU. We also aimed to gain a better understanding of the significance of parental participation in the care of children on NICUs, including factors that influence, facilitate or obstruct that participation. Our studies ended in three separate scientific papers (Wigert *et al.* 2006, Wigert *et al.* 2007, Wigert *et al.* 2008). In this chapter, we offer an outline of the insights from these three studies and an overall interpretative synthesis of our findings.

Methodology

We chose to carry out the studies using a lifeworld hermeneutic approach as described by Dahlberg *et al.* (2008; also refer to Dahlberg, Chapter 2). This offered a basis from which to analyse the world as experienced and communicated by people.

The philosophical idea of the lifeworld was introduced by Husserl (1970) and further developed by Merleau-Ponty (1995). The lifeworld is the every-day world in which we live our lives and take all our activities for granted. The lifeworld theory can be a basis for both a phenomenological and hermeneutical approach. Hermeneutic philosophy holds that the basis of understanding is being in the world and, consequently, the interpretation of that world and that language is an essential tool for understanding as it gives access to other people's experiences. This philosophy highlights pre-understand-ing as an intentional structure which is always activated when objects are regarded as something, and which forms the presupposition for understand-ing (Gadamer 1995) (also discussed by Smythe in Chapter 3). In lifeworld research the researcher should have an open and sensitive attitude towards the phenomenon being focused on, bridling their own pre-understandings through a distancing and reflective attitude to new experience (Dahlberg *et al.* 2008; refer also to Chapter 2). The intention is to be ready to see, inter-pret and understand something new in a new way (Gadamer 2004).

Ethical issues

The study setting for the enquiries was located in the western part of Sweden. We gained ethical approval and consent to undertake all the studies from the Local Research Ethics Committee. Verbal consent was obtained from the participants in each study after they had been given written and oral information that, among other issues, included the voluntariness of participation and the confidential treatment of all collected data.

Interviews and fieldwork

In our first two studies (Wigert *et al.* 2006, Wigert *et al.* 2007) we collected data through interviews. The essential feature of this research was the posing of open questions in order for the studied world to be explored and revealed. In each case, the interviews were started with an open question followed by clarifying questions such as: 'What do you mean?'; 'Can you describe further?'; 'Can you give an example?'. In the third study we used participative observations combined with clarifying interviews (Wigert *et al.* 2008). The observations were, like the interviews, directed at the studied phenomenon and gave access to interpersonal interactions. The combination of observations and interviews provided an insider's perspective on the phenomenon in its natural setting (Dahlberg *et al.* 2008).

Analysis

All collected data, both from interviews and observations, were transcribed into text. The analysis followed principles described by Dahlberg *et al.* who emphasize that a lifeworld hermeneutic approach in the analysis does not use any predetermined hypotheses, nor any theories or other interpretive sources. The focus for the analysis was on meanings in the text which were condensed, compared and grouped. In repeating readings of the text, clusters evolved and were sorted into sub-themes which were compared, contrasted and finally formed into themes. This work was followed with tentative interpretations of the themes of meaning in order to identify underlying conditions for the phenomena. Throughout the analysis an open and critical distanced and reflective reading of the text was used in order to uncover explanations. This means that openness and pliability was complemented with a distancing, and a reflective and critical approach. In order to decide whether there was a discrepancy between understanding of the parts and of the whole, interpretations of the parts were constantly compared with the interpretation of the whole. Finally all valid tentative interpretations were compared and synthesized resulting in a main interpretation (Dahlberg *et al.* 2008).

Findings

Study one: 'How do mothers experience having their newborn child in NICU?'

Ten tape-recorded interviews were performed with mothers in response to the first research question, 'how do mothers being cared for on the maternity ward experience having their child in NICU?' We decided to choose mothers of full-term children because premature children often have a more complex situation. The mothers were chosen strategically in that all had some distance from the event; this period ranged from six months to six years. The open question in the interviews was: 'Please, describe your experiences when your newborn child was cared for in a NICU during the postpartum period'. (For full details of the methodology see Wigert *et al.* 2006.)

The analysis illuminated that the mothers' feelings alternated between exclusion and participation, with the emphasis on exclusion. A feeling of exclusion was present when there had been a lack of interaction with the HCP. This implied a sense of not belonging to either the maternity care unit or the NICU, and appeared to have a negative effect on maternal identity. When a greater feeling of participation had been experienced this was combined with a continuous dialogue, feelings of being valued as a unique person with unique needs, and positive maternal feelings. Three themes were indentified:

- feeling of interaction
- feeling of belonging or not belonging
- maternal feelings.

Feeling of interaction

In the theme feeling of interaction the mothers' need for communication, information and trust was expressed. Verbal information was an important part of the interaction; however, there was often a lack of information provided by HCPs:

> I had no idea where my child was or who was caring for him. No, nobody told me.
>
> (Mother)

This led to speculation about what the HCPs were doing with the child in the mother's absence. A feeling of exclusion evolved. The mother wanted to get information and conversation with the HCPs about their child, but had to develop their own strategies to be informed:

> I learnt that the coffee room was at the end of the neonatal corridor, and that the doctor took a coffee break every morning at 9 o'clock. ... Then he couldn't go past without saying something.
>
> (Mother)

When continuous information was provided this led to trust in the HCP's knowledge and treatment. The trust included a feeling of being understood and treated as a unique mother with unique needs, as well as a feeling of trust of oneself at the time of leaving the hospital:

> They know how to deal with me, to keep me calm…the people who worked there [the maternity ward] also knew the neonatal ward so I received very good support, they took care of me.
>
> (Mother)

Feeling of belonging or not belonging

Another crucial theme was the feeling of belonging or not belonging. Most children were in hospital for more than a week. Simultaneously, the mothers received care in the maternity unit but expressed that they belonged neither to the maternity care unit nor to the NICU:

> I never met any of the staff [the maternity ward]; no I don't think I have spoken to anybody down there.
>
> (Mother)

The mothers felt that they had nothing in common with other mothers in the maternity ward who had their child with them. It was emotionally difficult to interact and engage with them, and, instead, they found fellowship with mothers who were in a similar situation.

In the NICU there was no bed or place for the mothers and there was a feeling of not being welcome. The rooms and surroundings were not welcoming and often it was impossible to find a place to be alone with their child:

> It didn't feel right being there [the neonatal ward] either. Nobody sent me away, but when he was asleep, I felt that I was intruding.
>
> (Mother)

Maternal feelings

The third theme was maternal feelings. The first meeting with the child was a crucial experience; a confirmation of 'being a whole woman', fortified as a mother. When the HCP in NICU cared for the child, feelings of powerlessness were frequent in the mother who was both tired after a difficult childbirth and filled with a guilty conscience for not taking care of her own child. The child was experienced as belonging more to the HCP than to the mothers themselves. Even the care the mother was capable of giving was taken over by the HCPs:

> They are experts in some way. You feel superfluous, they change [nappies] him, they are a lot more skilled, that was the feeling I had…they

> are real specialists of course but it's perhaps unnecessary. Perhaps I am
> not needed as a mother as they do it so much better.
>
> (Mother)

Since early pregnancy the mothers were repeatedly informed at the antenatal clinic that the first contact with the child after childbirth was essential. During the separation, several mothers experienced a feeling of not being a mother; intellectually they knew they were a mother but these maternal feelings were denied. A crucial question was if this early separation could influence their relationship with their child:

> I didn't feel that I had given birth to a child. It was not until he disappeared, and he was only up and turned over on my stomach, and then he was gone.
>
> (Mother)

Study two: 'How do health care professionals experience parental participation in NICU?'

The results from the previous study raised a new research question: 'how do health care professionals experience parents' presence and participation in the care of their child in the NICU?' Tape-recorded open interviews with 20 HCPs, four physicians, nine nurses and seven paediatric nurse assistants were performed. The HCPs worked at one of two NICUs; either at a University hospital or a county hospital in the same Swedish region. Two open questions were posed: 'How do you feel about parents participating in the care of their child in NICU?', and 'What do you do to facilitate that participation?' (For full details on the methodology employed in the study refer to Wigert *et al.* 2007.)

The NICU at the University hospital had 22 beds and a staff of 120 admitting seriously ill neonates from other regional hospitals, and having a high turnover of patients often leading to a heavy workload. The local NICU had 15 beds and a staff of 60. Both of the NICUs had intensive-care rooms, with one and two rooms for less intensive care, respectively. There were also parent rooms, which enabled a parent to stay alone or together with the child if its condition allowed. The University NICU had two parent rooms, and the local NICU had five.

The result of the analysis gave four tentative interpretations presented as four themes:

- to train parents in parenthood
- to use oneself
- participating parents both facilitate and obstruct care work
- the care environment both facilitates and obstructs.

To train parents in parenthood

HCPs expressed a responsibility for the whole family with the aim of care being to form a functional family with competent parents who had the prerequisites to deal with the strain at home. They saw themselves as experts in caring, who thereby knew the characteristics of a 'good parent'. The parents had to first show that they could take care of the child before they were allowed to take over responsibility:

> To guide the parents and make sure that they become parents is actually the most important job in the unit.
>
> (Nurse)

The HCPs seemed to function as gatekeepers, setting the limits for when and what the parents should be permitted to do with their child. An essential limit for parental participation was the condition of the child. They wanted to involve the parents in the care, but at the same time they wanted to carry out the care themselves as they knew how it should be done and they could do it faster. They also expressed concern about parents being too involved in the care of their child, taking over the carer's tasks:

> It is very important that the parents also understand what role they should take, set limits. Otherwise it is easy for the parents to take over, they start doing things they shouldn't.
>
> (Nurse)

To use oneself

This theme focuses the importance of how the HPCs used themselves in the encounter with the parents. This included the desire to satisfy the unique parent's needs and resources, and to find a balance between closeness and distance in this relationship. The extremes of how HCPs used themselves ranged from being very personal and sharing their own experiences, to putting up a front towards the parents. The relationships between HCPs and parents became closer when parents had particular needs, when the child was hospitalized for a longer period of time and when their relationship was felt to be harmonious.

From a HCP perspective, a central part of their role was to instil trust and hope. It was however difficult to meet parents when there were worries about the prognosis and when it was not possible for the mother to deliver a healthy child. Thus, when the parents were in greatest need, the HCPs found it most difficult to encounter them. One way to handle the situation was to avoid eye contact with the parents:

You can avoid eye contact, you can be asked questions that you don't really know how to answer or it takes too long and that is a characteristic you shouldn't have in neonatal care.

(Nurse)

Participating parents facilitate and obstruct care work

Another dimension in the HCPs' narratives was that participating parents were experienced as sometimes facilitating and sometimes obstructing the HCPs' work. Their presence and involvement was experienced as both an asset and an encumbrance. It was enriching to meet new unique parents who also could relieve some of the care workload:

We don't have the resources to take care of the child completely, it is built on the fact that the parents should take care of their child as well.

(Physician)

At the same time the parents' participation diminished the HCPs' opportunities to be on their own with the child or forced them to wait for tasks to be performed. Furthermore, being observed all the time by parents was felt to be tiring, though at the same time the carer knew that the parents' presence was important for the child:

You become tired sometimes, we are observed 7 out of 8 hours at work. You are judged and evaluated.

(Paediatric nurse assistant)

The care environment facilitates and obstructs

The care environment appeared both to facilitate and obstruct the HCPs' efforts to involve the parents in the care of their child. There seemed to be more obstacles concerning the facilities, in particular in one of the units. A main problem was that the rooms were not designed for the parents' needs, which the HCP tried to compensate for:

You try to screen off the parents so that they have a little corner for themselves and it is of great importance where in the room the child is placed. If you know that it is a bad situation with sad parents then you don't place them nearest to the door.

(Nurse)

A feeling of powerlessness was present among the HCPs and different opinions were expressed. They wanted a different model of care organization that addressed the needs of the whole family, both child and parents:

It would be good if there were more co-care wards where you could care for more mothers and children together...where they (parents) could be a little more involved.

(Physician)

HCPs also expressed a wish for their skills to be confirmed by the management. In the absence of this, they searched for affirmation from the parents:

Grateful parents, that's the reward, that's what we all live on, why we stay, I think. Some reward from somewhere else is non-existent.

(Physician)

Study three: The conditions for parents' participation in the care of their child in NICU

Due to some divergences between the two studies previously undertaken, we needed more knowledge about parental participation. We decided to perform a field study on the two NICUs. This included participative observations and clarifying interviews with parents and HCPs directed towards the phenomenon; 'conditions of parents' participation in the care of their child on NICUs, identifying both facilitating and obstructing factors'. The observations viewed interpersonal interactions, and was combined with interviews with parents, HCPS, and management staff, to provide an insider's perspective on the phenomenon in its natural settings (Dahlberg *et al.* 2008).

The fieldwork was carried out by HW over 64 hours during 22 different working shifts. The observations were carefully described in field notes and, where possible, were transcribed during the actual observation or immediately following it. The next step consisted of reading the field notes and recalling the observed behaviours with all its content and complexities and summarising this in written personal reflections. (For further details on the methodology employed in the study refer to Wigert *et al.* 2007.)

Four interpretative themes were identified:

- the care environment is dominated by medical technique
- the ward rounds focus on the medical diagnosis, while caring needs are disregarded
- participation is on the terms of staff and the activity
- participation is important, but the economy is the controlling factor.

The care environment is dominated by medical technique

Two aspects of the care environment emerged as central, both of which facilitated and hindered parents' participation in the care of their children. These were the layout of the care rooms with their medical-technical equipment, and the specialization of care. The technical equipment occupied a large area at each care place and the units were often crammed with technical equipment, parents and HCPs. The HCPs made efforts to make a private sphere for the child's family with screens or drawn curtains. However, the large number of people going through the ward prevented the parents from being undisturbed with their children.

The medical-technical care gave the environment a particular feature that signalled the care priorities. The equipment and staff that surrounded their child provided a visual clue as to why parents might have felt in the way of staff. Nonetheless, the parents appeared to become acclimatized to the environment, and, after a while they even started to operate like the staff, such as turning off alarms themselves. Views on whether this type of parent participation was good or bad were divided among the staff:

> The parents do a lot, even with the equipment, and that terrifies me. That they pull the cables apart... the first times they are there to care for their child, someone [HCP] might say, 'Yes you can take out these electrodes'. But that is when the staff is there; the next time the dad might turn off the alarm to the respirator.
>
> (Nurse)

The HCPs showed a high level of competence in emergency and intensive care of the child and appeared to prioritize this type of care over nursing care. Presence and participation by parents at the NICU seemed central, but the nature of the care environment made their involvement less important. The medical-technical care had a clear priority of supporting the survival and recovery of the children. However, its central profile meant that less obvious nursing care, such as emotional based support and involvement of parents, was marginalized, rather than instrumental and emotional based care being complementary parts of a holistic based care package. Therefore it appeared that the presence of and participation by parents was not considered to have as high a priority as the medical-technical aspects of the care:

> If you are interested in equipment, tubes and leads, that is high status. If you are interested in meeting people, conversation, maybe it hasn't got as high a status.
>
> (HCP on a management position)

The ward rounds focus on the medical diagnosis, while the caring needs are disregarded

The ward round played a central part in the care environment and reinforced the medical-technical emphasis on care. The discussion focused on the medical status of the child, while its nursing care needs were considered to varying degrees. At one of the units, parents were not allowed to be present during the ward round, despite the fact that management staff thought their inclusion could be positive. This exclusion created unnecessary worry for the parents:

> At the time of the round, there was a total ban on entering the ward, and then you wonder as a parent why you can't listen when it is a ward round for your child?
>
> (Mother)

At the other unit parents were invited and encouraged to take part in the ward round. They were seen as a valuable resource that could contribute information about their child and the physicians were able to save time as they could inform the parents directly of the medical state and care of their child. This seemed to ease parental worries.

At both units the parents were not routinely formally briefed after the ward round. This led to many questions remaining unanswered. Individual parent–physician talks on the state of the child were seldom arranged at other times, and, when they did happen, they were often instigated at the parents' own initiative.

Participation is on the terms of the staff and the activity

The third theme focuses on the attitudes of the HCPs and the effect of this on the parents' capacity to participate in the care of their child at the NICU. During their stay in the maternity ward the mothers' opportunities to attend the NICU, and to leave when they wanted to, were related both to their own medical condition, and mostly (except when the child's father was present) based on HCPs' availability to accompany them. Parents returning to the NICU were usually told by the HCPs what had happened to their child since they were last there. Unfortunately, there were also shortcomings. Some parents' wishes were ignored or even overridden. For example, in some cases they were initially invited to participate and then they were later not being given the opportunity to do so if it did not fit in with the clinical activities of the ward:

> The parents are with their 5-day-old child, the mother for the second time, and the paediatric nurse assistant asks them: 'Should I show you how to cup feed him and then you can do it yourselves?' She lifts the sleeping child and is about to start feeding him when the ward round enters the ward. The parents are shown into the corridor and the paediatric nurse assistant cup feeds the child. The child is put to bed, the ward round finishes and the parents come in. They go to their child and ask: 'Is he going to eat?' The paediatric nurse assistant replies: 'He has had some, exemplary baby. He ate by himself, really good, it

went straight down.' The parents go up to the child's bed and lift the cover. The paediatric nurse assistant says: 'He is sleeping now, so we'll let him sleep.' The parents sit down beside the bed but cannot see their child as the canopy is drawn and leave the unit after a couple of minutes.

(Observation)

These observations revealed that the professional role of the HCPs was more consultative towards the parents. However, questions were also raised about this new role:

The parents have a natural, prominent role, but what is our role?

(Nurse)

Procedures used to find out why a mother was absent or documenting the presence of parents did not exist. Many shifts could pass with no attempt being made to find out the reason for the parents' absence. This conflict of wanting to demand greater parent participation, a lack of routines for documenting the presence of parents and, at the same time, uncertainty about which demands could be made and how much involvement there should be in the family's social situation seemed to be an obstacle to parents' participation in the care of their child.

Participation is important, but the economy is the controlling factor

The fourth theme describes the management's views on the parents' participation in the care of their child at the NICU. There was a high level of awareness of the importance of parental involvement. It was seen as a responsibility to promote an approach to care based on respect for the needs of the parents and parental participation. However, tangible guidelines as to how this should be done were lacking. A necessary condition of developing neonatal intensive care was for different categories of HCP to be working to achieve this goal, but in practice this was not the case. One reason was considered to be the difficulty of bringing together all the professional groups, with the physician group often being absent:

We must create the conditions to allow them to participate and that means we must be able to offer the parents the chance to be here.

(Management position)

Another pattern noted by the management staff was how the HCPs started from the perspective of their own needs when discussing care routines debilitating the development of NICU care:

Sometimes I have a feeling that we forget we are here for the patient, for the parents, maybe we are more used to thinking about ourselves, putting ourselves first.

(Management position)

Initiatives for getting parents to participate in their child's care had been introduced on the units. One was so-called 'parental training', during which nurses would talk to parents as a group about different topics, such as what it means to be a parent of a child at a NICU. However, an identified obstacle for drawing up strategies to promote parents' participation in the care of their child was the economic conditions set by the politicians:

Having a balanced economy is the most important thing, as long as patient safety can be guaranteed. We are the implementers, but the politicians who decide what should be done with the tax payers' money; they represent the people.

(Management position)

Main interpretation of parental participation at NICU: a synthesis of three studies

During a pregnancy, a relationship between the woman and her child develops. She prepares for motherhood and imagines how the first encounter with her child should be. When her newborn child needs extra care in a NICU, she finds herself in a situation for which she is unprepared. She is filled with different kinds of feelings during the separation, such as fear, guilt, anxiety, loneliness and a sense of not belonging. In this situation the interactions between the mother and the HCPs are important for her understanding of what is happening to her child. When she stays in the maternity ward while her child is in the NICU, insecurity occurs and a feeling of exclusion evolves for the mother. She belongs neither to the maternity care unit nor to the NICU. This feeling of exclusion is strengthened by difficulties in receiving care from the caregivers in the maternity care unit, having other mothers with a child beside them, and when not being seen as part of her child's care by HCPs on the NICU. When staff do not acknowledge the mother and her personal needs, this is understood as an uncaring behaviour impacting upon the dignity of the mother, which in turn leads to suffering. On the other hand, feelings of participation evolve when the mother is seen as a unique person with unique needs; involved as a natural part of her child's daily care, trying to breastfeed, or just being nearby if illness prevents other activities. This seems to positively influence maternal feelings of trustfulness in their sense of motherhood.

The conditions for parents to participate in the care of their child in NICU as described in this synthesis reveal many contradictions regarding visions and goals and the prevailing reality of care. Both management and HCPs had high ambitions to develop care that promotes parent partici-pation. In theory, they knew how they ought to behave, but observations showed that parents had limited opportunities to be active in the care. Ambivalence and limit setting for parents' participation were observed. The HCPs wanted to strengthen the parents' self-confidence, and encour-age them to develop their own routines in the care of the child. At the same time they acted as gate-keepers, restricting parental participation in several ways.

Another contradictory aspect was the HCP's expectations. On one hand, it was expected that parents should be present and participate in their child's care, whereas on the other hand they expressed hesitancy and insecurity about finding out the reasons for the parents' absence. It was apparent that the HCPs' roles were in a transition from performing all care for the child to doing it in collaboration with parents. It was a challenge to find a professional role that is governed by cooperation with the participat-ing parents, and not to see the parents in this partnership as competitors in the care of the child. A further obstacle was that the HCPs highlighted difficulties in engaging with worried parents, meeting their concerns and instilling trust and hope. It seemed that HCPs were often not able to cor-rectly deal with parents in crises.

A further barrier for parental participation was that nursing care, which includes the development of reliable, supporting relationships with parents, was subordinated to medical-technical aspects of care. The care environment also seemed to obstruct efforts to involve the parents in the care of their child. There was lack of space for parents, a short-age of HCPs, and, at one of the units, recurrent overcrowding. Another obstacle was the ward round, where the parents in one of the units were prohibited from being present, and where there was a pervasive difficulty in communicating with physicians. HCPs in a management capacity, from those with section responsibility to those with operational responsibility at an overall level, expressed the view that the goal was to promote presence and participation by parents. This too was contradicted when it was set against the economic resources that were a deciding force in the develop-ment of care at the unit.

Reflections on the results

This synthesis of our three lifeworld studies has shown that parents' par-ticipation in the care of their child in NICU is complex and influenced by obstacles and contradictions. The interpretative phase will be finalized through connecting the results to the wider existing literature.

Exclusion or participation?

It is well known that early contact during babyhood promotes maternal attachment to the child (Bowlby 1969, Ainsworth 1973, Klaus and Kennell 1982). However, to start motherhood by establishing a close relationship with a child who has been cared for in a NICU is a difficult task (Jackson *et al.* 2003). Our first study showed that the mothers altered between exclusion and participation (Wigert *et al.* 2006). As described by other researchers (Heerman *et al.* 2005) a feeling that the child belonged to the hospital arose. If denied the opportunity to mother their child, confusion and anxiety can worsen the parental situation (Fenwick *et al.* 2001, Lupton and Fenwick 2001).

Mothers in our studies had a desire and a right to be with their child, but most did not dare to exert force to attain their rights. The feelings of exclusion when the mother's own needs were not met led to a deep and embedded sense of loneliness. This was exacerbated by the personal suffering they endured due to their child's condition. To deny the mother's right to her own child is, according to Eriksson, an uncaring form of power, and an abuse (Eriksson 1997). For caring to exist at NICUs the HCPs must have courage and take responsibility for the mother of the child, ensuring that this suffering does not arise and that maternal participation dominates the care regimes. Negative effects arising from the separation of mother and child can be counteracted. Research has found that a mother who receives extra contact with her child shows greater commitment, has a higher level of self-esteem, and a greater knowledge in the interpretation of the child's signals (Lawhon 2002, Davis *et al.* 2003, Loo *et al.* 2003, Fegran *et al.* 2006).

Who owns the baby and who is allowed to care?

Our studies showed that parents were not given sufficient prerequisites to take their responsibility for taking care of their child as prescribed in policy documents (Föräldrabalken 1949: 381). The HCPs set limits for parental participation, and the children 'belonged' more to the ward than to the parents. Simultaneously, the HCPs showed ambivalence in parental participation. When there was a shortage of staff, the parents' participation reduced their workload, but their presence for the HCPs also meant being constantly observed and having comments on their work. This finding concurs with other studies (Fenwick *et al.* 2001, Lupton and Fenwick 2001, Heerman *et al.* 2005, Fegran and Helseth 2008).

The lack of participation was also shown in the routines in relation to the ward rounds at one of the studied NICUs. Parents' acceptance at being dismissed into the corridor may well reflect their position of dependence in the NICU. The result is similar to other research into parental participation in the paediatric care context (Hallström *et al.* 2002, Corlett and Twycross 2006, Ygge 2007).

Difficulty in meeting the parents

The research also highlights the need of a good relationship to be developed between the parents and HCPs in the care of a sick or prematurely born child. It was apparent that the carers saw themselves as experts in caring, but it is also important for HCPs to support the parents in the caring of their newborn. We believe that the person who knows most about which kind of support he/she needs is the parent himself/herself. To use words of philosopher Lögstrup (1997), 'in order to help another person, we must let the person himself/herself decide what is most helpful', i.e., give the parent the opportunity to decide what he/she wishes to participate in.

The difficulties for the HCPs to meet the worried parents and only see themselves as ordinary 'fellow men' are noteworthy. One way to behave when confronted with the parents' worry was avoidance, for example, avoiding eye contact with the parents. This observation led us to the work of the philosopher Sartre (2003), who has stated that people can make themselves adversaries to themselves in a difficult situation, by avoiding that situation. People become hostile and self-obliterating through this process. This might be a risk for professional carers who avoid engagement with difficult circumstances. To be a professional carer in NICU should by definition also include being able to meet parents in crisis.

Another prominent task for the HCPs that emerged from the findings relates to the necessity to instil hope and give comfort to the parents. To have hope is an essential and supreme motivational power of life which is nurtured in human relations, and there is considerable strength in instilling hope to others (Lögstrup 1997); it can both ease suffering and transform suffering into faith, courage and trust (Eriksson 1997).

The caring environment and advanced technology

A significant obstacle for the parents was the separation from the child and the limited possibilities to stay together with and be alone with their child. This illuminated how policies were not fulfilled (UNICEF 1989, NOBAB 1992). It is documented that significant distress can arise when no opportunity of being alone exists (Eriksson 1997). The care environment's failings in these aspects caused an unnecessary suffering for the HCPs as well. Even they needed to be able to withdraw and not always be exposed to the parents' observations and comments.

An ethical dilemma that evolved from the findings is that the medico-technical aspects of care were supervalued over nursing care. One reason for this may be that, in contemporary hospital-based health systems, it is completely unthinkable, and can also be punishable, to put aside medical-technical care; however, the consequences of putting aside nursing care appear unclear.

Methodological reflections

The use of a lifeworld approach, including data collection through open interviews and observations, offered possibilities to describe and understand the studied phenomena. In the interviews with the mothers a long period had passed since the event (six months to six years). Despite this, it was surprising how vivid and emotional the experiences of separation were. Once the interviews started the narratives just flowed and were told with great detail and enthusiasm (Wigert *et al.* 2006). This demonstrated how important the experience was, and that it remained with the mothers for a long period of time. Even the HCPs' stories (Wigert *et al.* 2007) were strongly emotional. One HCP cried, whilst others demonstrated anger, or were exhausted during the interviews.

To combine the interviews with observations was important, albeit challenging, especially when some of the more negative phenomena were viewed through the observer's eyes. It is well known that if the researching observer is an expert in the area being studied, which was the case for HW as a neonatal nurse, there is a risk he/she will forget the role as an observer and act like a nurse. During data collection HW constantly strived to bridle her own pre-understanding and to focus on the studied phenomenon (Dahlberg *et al.* 2008).

During the analyses of the texts in all the studies, we constantly reflected on how our respective pre-understandings influenced the interpretations. An objective understanding was not possible, but the cooperation between us was an asset in the process (Gadamer 2004) to understand more about the meaning of parents' participation in the care of their child in a NICU.

Conclusion and practical implications

According to current policies in Sweden the parents are welcomed to stay with and participate in the care of their newborn child when it needs care in a NICU. Our study shows that the personnel had good ambitions to develop ideal care that promoted parent participation. However, care mainly seemed to be driven by budget constraints and medical-technical aspects; and parental participation was on the terms of the staff who had difficulty in meeting worried parents.

Although these studies are performed in a Swedish context we believe there is a core of meanings that could be generalized to other NICUs in other countries. These results highlight that there is need to develop tangible strategies that provide optimal conditions for the parent to be present and involved in the care of their child on a NICU. This includes defining staff guidelines on working with families. Further it includes training HCPs in the art of encountering and dealing with parents in crisis; which can be done in organized groups where the participants in a safe and calm environment permit reflection on their own actions and attitudes to parents.

References

Adshead G. and Bluglass K. (2005) Attachment representations in mothers with abnormal illness behaviour by proxy. *British Journal of Psychiatry* 187, 328–333.

Ainsworth M.D.S. (1973) The development of infant–mother attachment. In: *Review of Child Development Research, 3* (eds B.M. Caldwell and H.N Ricciuti), 41–93. Chicago University of Press: Chicago.

Bowlby J. (1969) *Attachment and Loss. Volume 1.* Basic Books: New York.

Cescutti-Butler L. and Galvin K. (2003) Parents' perceptions of staff competency in a neonatal intensive care unit. *Journal of Clinical Nursing* 12, 752–761.

Corlett J. and Twycross A. (2006) Negotiation of parental roles within family-centred care: a review of the research. *Journal of Clinical Nursing* 15, 1308–1316.

Dahlberg K., Dahlberg H. and Nyström M. (2008) *Reflective Lifeworld Research.* Studentlitteratur: Lund.

Davis L., Mohay H. and Edwards H. (2003) Mothers' involvement in caring for their premature infants: an historical overview. *Journal of Advanced Nursing* 42, 578–586.

Eriksson K. (1997) Understanding the world of the patient, the suffering being: the new clinical paradigm from nursing to caring. *Advanced Practicing Nursing Quarterly* 3, 8–13.

Fegran L. and Helseth S. (2008) The parent–nurse relationship in neonatal intensive care unit context: closeness and emotional involvement. *Scandinavian Journal of Caring Sciences* 14, Epub.

Fegran L., Helseth S., Slettebø Å. (2006) Nurses as moral practitioners encountering parents in neonatal intensive care units. *Nursing Ethics* 13, 52–64.

Fenwick J., Barclay L. and Schmeid V. (2001) Struggling to mother: a consequence of inhibitive nursing interactions in the neonatal nursery. *Journal of Perinatal Neonatal Nursing* 15, 49–64.

Föräldrabalken (1949:381) (Swedish Children and Parents Code). Available at: http://www.notisum.se/rnp/SLS/lag/19490381.htm [Accessed 6 February 2010].

Franck L.S. and Spencer C. (2003) Parent visiting and participations in infant care giving activities in a neonatal unit. *Birth* 30, 31–35.

Gadamer H-G. (1995) *Truth and Method.* 2nd edn (Trans. J. Weinsheimer and D. Marshall). The Continuum Publishing Company: New York.

Gadamer H-G. (2004) *Truth and Method.* 3rd edn. Continuum: New York.

Griffin T. and Abraham M. (2006) Transition to home from the newborn intensive care unit: applying the principles of family-centered care to the discharge process. *Journal of Perinatal Neonatal Nursing* 20, 243–249.

Hallström I., Runeson I. and Elander G. (2002) An observational study of the level at which parents participate in decisions during their child's hospitalization. *Nursing Ethics* 9, 202–214.

Heerman J., Wilson M. and Wilhelm P. (2005) Mothers in the NICU: outsider to partner. *Pediatric Nursing* 31,176–181.

Husserl E. (1970) *Logical investigations: Vol 1. Prolegomena to pure logic.* (Trans. J. Findlay) (Orig: Logische Undtersuchhungen). Routledge Kegan Paul: London.

Jackson K., Ternestedt B-M. and Scollin J. (2003) From alienation to familiarity: experiences of mothers and fathers of preterm infants. *Journal of Advanced Nursing* 43, 120–129.

Kennell J. and McGrath S. (2005) Starting the process of mother–infant bonding. *Acta Paeditric* 94, 775–777.

Klaus M.H. and Kennell J.H. (1982) *Parent–Infant Bonding*. Mosby: St Louis.

Lawhon G. (2002) Facilitation of parenting the premature infant within the newborn intensive care unit. *Journal of Perinatal Neonatal Nursing* 16, 71–82.

Lögstrup K.E. (1997) *The Ethical Demand*. (Original work published 1956). University of Notre Dame Press: USA.

Loo K.K., Espinosa M., Tyler R. and Howard J. (2003) Using knowledge to cope with stress in the NICU: how parents integrate learning to read the physiologic and behavioural cues of the infant. *Neonatal Network* 22, 31–37.

Lupton D. and Fenwick J. (2001) They've forgotten that I'm the mum: constructing practising motherhood in special care nurseries. *Social Science and Medicine* 53, 1011–1021.

Merleau Ponty M. (1995/1945) *Phenomenology of Perception*. Routledge: London.

Nordic Association for Sick Children in Hospital (NOBAB 1992) Nordic standard for care of children and adolescents in hospital. Available at: http://www.nobab.se [Accessed 6 February 2010].

Sartre J-P. (2003) *Being and Nothingness*. Taylor & Francis: Oxford.

United Nations Convention on the Rights of the Child. (UNICEF 1989). Available at: http://www.unicef.org/crc/commitment.htm [Accessed 6 February 2010].

Wigert H., Johansson R., Berg M. and Hellström A-L. (2006) Mothers' experiences of having their newborn child in a neonatal intensive care unit. *Scandinavian Journal of Caring Sciences* 20, 35–41.

Wigert H., Berg M. and Hellström A-L. (2007) Health care professionals' experiences of parental presence and participation in neonatal intensive care unit. *International Journal of Qualitative Studies on Health and Well-being* 2, 45–54.

Wigert H., Hellström A-L. and Berg M. (2008) Conditions for parents' participation in the care of their newborn child in a neonatal intensive care – a field study. *BioMEd Central Pediatrics* 23, 8: 3.

Ygge B-M. (2007) Nurses' perceptions of parental involvement in hospital care. *Paediatric Nursing* 17, 38–40.

10 A poetic hermeneutic phenomenological analysis of midwives 'being with woman' during childbirth

Lauren P. Hunter

Introduction

The profession of midwifery in the United States considers therapeutic presence an essential part of midwifery care (ACNM 2004). In this chapter I present the findings of a hermeneutical phenomenological exploration of the meaning of 'being with woman' for a specific group of American midwives. These interpretations have been elucidated through poetry written by American midwives about being a midwife or attending women in childbirth. I have used poetry as the basis of interpretation due to the power of poetic metaphor to provide a rich source of unique human meaning, suited to qualitative enquiry (Hunter 2002a).

The importance of 'being with woman' for the midwifery profession

Research has revealed that women-centred care and 'being with woman' are important (Callister and Freeborn 2007). Hunter (2002b) defined 'being with woman' as 'the provision of emotional, physical, spiritual, and psychological support by the midwife as desired by the labouring woman' (p. 615). Furthermore, a previous hermeneutical phenomenological study by Hunter (2008) discovered three ways of midwifery knowing: self, grounded, and informed, which were integral components in the provision of midwifery care and 'being with woman' (see Figure 10.1 on page 175).

A plethora of qualitative studies have demonstrated that women and midwives value the midwifery care concept of 'being with woman', especially during childbirth (for example, Berg 2005, Sjoblom *et al.* 2006, Bayes *et al.* 2008, John 2009, Lundgren *et al.* 2009). 'Being with woman' has also been linked to positive outcomes for childbearing women, such as increased feeling of control and confidence during childbirth (Lundgren 2005, Fahy and Parratt 2006) and fewer negative childbirth memories (Lundgren 2005, Waldensttrom *et al.* 2006). Studies of American midwifery's theoretical framework have also included this concept as an essential hallmark of midwifery care (Cragin 2004).

Poetry as data for interpretation

Poetry is an excellent source for new meaning and understanding of tangible, poorly understood, or difficult to quantify concepts because it emanates from lived human experience, is aesthetic, evocative, and understandable across time and culture. Readers of poetry have the ability to understand and 'feel' a poem as they interpret the lived experience through the written word of the poet's conscious and unconscious mind.

Gadamer (1989) believed written language, such as poetry, provided a unique opportunity for interpretation of the present through the past. He thought language was fundamental to our being in the world and our interpretation of it, because it gave expression to all reasoning and all thoughts. Van Manen (1997) believed poetry was free from conventional style and capable of expressing intense feelings of linguistic expression for interpretation. Poetry's contribution to the nursing profession, patient care, and nursing research has been previously described in Hunter (2002a) and Hunter (2003).

Methodology

Hunter's (2000) anthology of poetry was a source for some of the poems used within this chapter. Other sources of poetry were the internet, published poetry books, and multiple library database searches using the keywords 'poetry', 'poems', 'childbirth' and 'midwifery'. Inclusion criteria for the poems were that they were written by an American midwife and were about attending a woman during childbirth or the experience of being a midwife. Written permission to use each poem was received prior to the study. A final sample of 18 from a total of 210 possible poems was eligible for interpretation as they directly referred to the lived experience of a midwife 'being with woman'.

Dilthey's (1987) human science philosophy, which stressed the importance of subjective information gathered textually as a unique opportunity to gain meaning about human experiences, and Gadamer's (1989) philosophical tenants guided this qualitative hermeneutic phenomenological study. Gadamer's (1989) hermeneutical circle was initiated by myself, as an active participant, to explore back and forth from self to the text for interpretation with a new meaning. The hermeneutical circle required the belief that prior biases and motivations influenced understanding, and that the aim was not to finally understand the truth, but to understand differently. The van Manen human science research method (1997), using four research activities specific for data analysis, was used for this study (also described by Dowling, Chapter 4). The research activities were not sequential, but instead I moved in a dynamic back and forth fashion among the activities. The first activity required 'turning to a phenomenon of interest'. The interest in 'being with woman' and poetry as data occurred because of my pre-understandings, assumptions, and definition of self based upon my culture and society: a midwife, nurse, mother, poet, and researcher. Gadamer (1989) believed that one's historical perspective and understandings could not be set aside in order to prevent contamination, but instead needed to be embraced and acknowledged as important to a hermeneutical interpretation.

The second research activity, 'investigating experience as we live it', allowed me to use my 'tacit-priori' experience as a midwife and the personal lived experiences of midwives' poetry to explore 'being with woman'. Third, I used self-reflection and van Manen's (1997) three-level approach to examine the poems as whole, via verse and metaphor and finally individual lines of poetry to identify the essential themes. Further development of themes occurred as I wrote interpretive sentences and narrative text, back and forth between my pre-understandings of 'being with woman' and the poems to develop a narrative text that portrayed the essential themes.

Draper's (1996) criterion for evaluation was used to judge the confirmability of the study. Three expert midwives verified the plausibility (credibility) of the themes and content authentication of 'being with woman' that emerged from the poetry. After reviewing the poetry data set and my narrative interpretation, each expert was asked to answer, 'Can you see in the written text my interpretation of "being with woman" and believe it?' Their positive responses indicated the authenticity of the interpretations and transferability of the themes. Audibility was achieved as my thought processes during theme development were documented in a research journal maintained throughout the study and evidenced by the sequential written drafts of my interpretations.

Findings

The interpretive phenomenological analysis from my original study (Hunter 2008) uncovered three essential themes: (a) 'experienced guidance'; (b) 'spiritual connections'; and (c) 'partners in birth'. Additional analysis of the 18 poems identified a number of sub-themes, which subsequently formed the basis of my interpretations of 'being with woman' (Figure 10.1). For illustrative purposes, poetic exemplars are *italicized* and embedded in the text for discussion of findings.

Experienced guidance

Experienced guidance was the most salient theme of 'being with woman' that was uncovered through the poetic interpretations. It was the art and act of guiding the woman through the labour and birth process carried out by the midwife. The sub-themes that emerged from this additional analysis were: (a) providing safety and protection; (b) embodied power; (c) reading

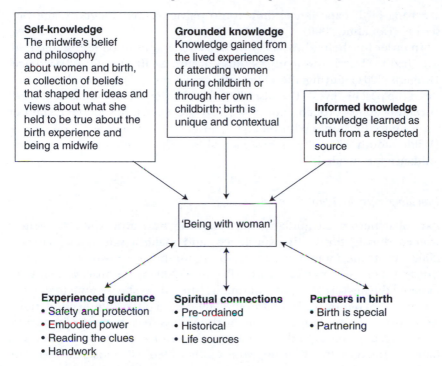

Figure 10.1 Diagrammatic representation of 'being with woman'.

the clues; and (d) handwork. Experienced guidance was knowing what to do: 'I spread a web gossamer like and strong as steel, I spin a safe place for her' (Wildermouth 2000); or what not to do, 'knowing when to be silent' (Bowen 2000b); how to do it, 'adept, sensing precisely balancing pressure and release' (Whitson 2000); and when it needed to be done, she 'summoned your mother to the one strong knot that would hold and secure. Your baby needs you now India...' (Brendsel 2000a).

Experienced guidance included grounded knowledge because the woman had shared and participated in many birth experiences: 'experienced midwife's hands, where baby upon baby landed' (Brendsel 2000b), and or because of her personal birth experience(s): I 'remember my children's birth' (Van Gorder 2000). In these accounts, the poets recounted their understanding of the nuances of labour, including the physical sensations: 'labor grips her in hands of steel' (Wildermouth 2000), and how women responded emotionally to labour: 'she sinks into herself...travelling in a world removed, and altered state' (Whitson 2000), and to birth: 'she reached down, drawing her daughter to her breast' (Walsh 1993). The poems suggest that experienced guidance also required a repertoire of expert skills based on informed knowledge to ensure a safe and satisfying birth experience: 'how to do pelvic exams...diagnose and pre-scribe' (Donahue 2000).

In order for the midwife's knowledge and actions to be useful, the mid-wife had to 'be with woman', because 'I have a gift, the gift of presence' (Roberts 2001) during the childbirth experience. Through observation: 'tears slip past her eyes' (Brendsel 2000a), voice: 'over and over she chanted' (Brendsel 2000a), touch: 'our hands...strong against her tailbone counter pressure to the pain' (Whitson 2000), and listening: 'moans become cries' (Wildermouth 2000), the midwife was able to determine whether and how guidance was needed.

Providing safety and protection

Part of experienced guidance was knowing how and when to protect women during the birth experience 'and make a safe place' (Parker 2000). Protection was vital during labour and birth for two reasons. First, 'those in her care are vulnerable' (Brendsel 2000b) because women were exposed during birth, both emotionally, 'she thinks she is going to die, she has no will of her own' (Wildermouth 2000), and physically. Second, there were also inherent dangers in the birth process that the midwife must be knowledgeable about and guard against to ensure safety for mother and baby, 'in the dark that morning your mother bled' (Brendsel 2000a). The midwife provided safety and protection as a proactive measure to prevent dangerous events from occurring in the first place because she was 'being with woman... I stand over her offering protection' (Wildermouth 2000), and keeping vigil knowing when to 'act swiftly, protecting life' (Bowen 2000b).

Embodied power

The midwife poets believed that women can and do successfully give birth, 'being at the woman's side who gathers from in her self the power to bear this new person into the light' (Whitson 2000). They knew that a woman's body, mind, and spirit were strong and capable of birth: 'a primal image majestic in her strength' (Wildermouth 2000).

> This woman, the round circles of her body
> All her forces concentrating
> On the work of this birth
>
> (Whitson 2000)

Through 'being with woman', the poets saw themselves as being able to assist and encourage women to give birth with the power and resources of their own bodies. They write about how they inspire power in the woman by telling her how well she was doing, 'You're almost there, You're doing so beautifully' (Walsh 1993), or with a simple gesture of her hand, 'soft on her arm for comfort and confidence' (Whitson 2000). They actively enhanced the woman's feeling of power through the use of powerful messages about her own strength and belief in herself: 'you are so strong' (Walsh 1993); 'you can do this and believing it' (Bowen 2000b).

In addition, the writers knew that women had an unconscious, historical knowing about birth, 'feeling the power of my own body doing what women's powerful bodies have always done' (Van Gorder 2000), that allowed them to trust their body to do the work of birth. They also used historical reminders of women who had laboured before to inspire confidence and strength, 'there's a woman in the mountain laboring, there's a woman in the ocean laboring, there's a woman in the jungle laboring and you can labor too' (Kalman 2000).

Reading the clues

Reading the clues described the delicate balance a midwife required while 'being with woman' so that she knew when to intervene and assist the woman through the birth process and when to leave her alone, and provide watchful waiting (a judgement that is also reported by Lundgren in Chapter 7). This was the continuous dynamic process of 'being with woman' that dictated what was done or not done to provide experienced guidance. By 'being with woman', the midwife was able to read the clues correctly.

Clue reading required that the midwife, as an experienced guide, be competent and knowledgeable about the labour and birth process, 'all is well, progressing nicely; we shall see this baby by noon' (Bowen 2000a). Through the act of reading clues correctly the midwife knew how labour was progressing, 'nagging pain, low in the belly starts to rise and fall in patterns faster, stronger' (Wildermouth 2000), or her expression as it changed from 'excitement, to concentration' (Walsh 1993), and how the woman was responding to labour, 'I know that you are frightened' (Kalman 2000). Based on the midwife's interpretation of the clues she decided to either do something: 'I will hold your hands and cry with you' (Roberts 2001), or continued 'watchful waiting': 'I sit near, I watch' (Wildermouth 2000). Because the midwife was part of the lived experience of each woman's unique childbirth, the midwife poets reported that she was able to interpret the clues correctly.

Handwork

The midwife's hands were the most conspicuous and important physical manifestation of self as an instrument of experienced guidance for the birth experience:

My hands
have measured and timed
examined, supported
comforted, held...
have touched new life
have guided and welcomed it
into the world

(Trout 2000)

Part of experienced guidance through handwork was knowing where, when, and how to touch 'our hands working with her' (Whitson 2000) to provide comfort and reassurance: 'I will hold your hands' (Kalman 2000). 'Hands, these hands, my hands, a midwife's hands' (Trout 2000) had a symbolic meaning for midwifery. The midwife's hands were one part of a trilogy of tangible circles present at the culmination of birth. The three actual circles were the midwife's hands that encircled the perineum as she assisted in the birth, 'our hands on the emerging circle' (Whitson 2000), the vagina that became a large circle to accommodate the coming head, 'one last push over a glistening perineum' (Bowen 2000a), and the baby's round head, 'the disc of dark hair becomes the crown of life' (Wildermouth 2000), as it was born into hands of the midwife. The midwife's experienced hands were the physical bridge that guided the newborn between before life and present life, 'teetering long between the blessed worlds' (Perdomo 2000c), and between life and death 'as new life approaches, always in company with the spectre of death' (Bowen 2000a).

   In the poems, the midwife was usually the first person to actually touch the newborn as she assisted in the woman's birth: 'I hold out my hands and touch the warm moist head' (Wildermouth 2000). She used her hands in the finals moments of labour to provide support to the perineum and make sure the baby's head was born slowly and gently, 'like a birthday balloon filled with dark hair and a flattened nose' (Perdomo 2000d). The midwife's competent hands helped to prevent the mother's perineum from tearing, and ensured a safe birth, 'born so smoothly in your shiny bubble you were protected from harm until in fact you had arrived' (Perdomo 2000d), that was also gentle for the newborn: 'love's touch...in the palm of her hand' (Parker 2000). The midwife's hands in the final moments assisted the newborn into its new world: 'midwives' hands working sure, guiding you, rotating you into the world' (Perdomo 2000c).

   In emergency situations the midwife had to be able to think and act competently; the 'midwife moved her hands quickly' (Brendsel 2000a). For instance, in one poem the midwife used her hands to stimulate an unresponsive baby to breathe by rubbing it with a warm cloth on its back and extremities, 'there limp in my hands, needed rubs and jump starts' (Brendsel 2000b). If manual stimulation and oxygen were not success-ful, 'as trembling hands work to hold, to touch and disturb you into life'

(Perdomo 2000a), then the midwife had to begin resuscitation, 'moved beat upon beat towards your heart' (Perdomo 2000a).

In the poetry, through experienced guidance, the midwife's hands ensured that the circle and mystery of life were successful: 'the cycle repeats itself and the mystery remains' (Bowen 2000b).

Spiritual connections

A spiritual connection was an essential theme that first appeared through the spiritual nature of many words found in the poetry such as souls, spirit, miracles, prayer, and God. Reflection upon the poetry revealed three sub-themes of spiritual connections (a) pre-ordained connections; (b) historical connections; and (c) life source connections. Spiritual connections helped to guide the midwife to 'being with woman' during childbirth.

As a part of self- knowledge, the midwife understands that she was meant to be a midwife; 'I remember in my cells' (Van Gorder 2000), before it becomes a conscious decision on her part, 'I have known the emotional work since before I was born' (Roberts 2001). The midwife knows that it is a special calling and preordained destiny, 'a part of life's plan' (Parker 2000), to be with women in childbirth. As part of the midwife's grounded knowledge, her belief is that her calling is special, she is meant to work in the profession of midwifery: 'we have always done this' (Whitson 2000), and is particularly suited to the work of midwifery.

For these poets, the midwife's self-knowledge allows her to recognize that women have cared for birthing women since the beginning of time, 'this work we have done all the length of history' (Whitson 2000), through a historical perspective, 'history is only our conscious memory' (Whitson 2000). The midwife knows that historically women have always been able to give birth, 'women's bodies knowing how to give birth' (Van Gorder 2000). The midwife believed in the sanctity of birth, 'it is a sacred mystery ancient and ever blessed' (Perdomo 2000b) and that it was an essence of midwifery, 'it is a covenant sealed upon the midwives soul' (Perdomo 2000b).

Because midwives believe in a spiritual source of power that is able to work through her, she actively sought assistance from that source in times of need, 'without words she called that other source' (Brendsel 2000a). In addition, the midwife recognized that there was more to a successful and safe birth experience, a 'prayer for safe passage' (Bowen 2000a), than just the midwife's skills and competence based upon her knowledge. The midwife believed that there was an imperceptible part of labour and birth that she ultimately could not control, 'daily miracles' (Trout 2000), and there was something greater than herself that had power in the universe. The midwife respected and revered this source of spirituality and called upon it to work through her as she routinely practised her profession and in times of great need.

Pre-ordained connections

In the poems, entering the profession of midwifery was likened to that of a spiritual calling, 'a calling it's called' (Laminack 2000). The midwife knew that she had been chosen to become a midwife, 'it found me, God gave me a gift' (Roberts 2001); even though at first she might not have been sure exactly what kind of gift she had been given: 'some without even a clear understanding why' (Laminack 2000).

However, when a midwife understood her inner spiritual source, 'the path lies before me' (Parker 2000) and accepted the preordained calling to become a midwife, she did so because of the personal beliefs that shaped her self-knowledge and her ideas about how birth was experienced, 'laughing shouting, crying – all the emotions of birth' (Walsh 1993), and how she, as a midwife, honours birth as a normal process, 'to help a sister bring forth a child in as loving and gentle way as I know how' (Laminack 2000). A midwife accepted the call and became a midwife because she knew she could make a difference for women and their families in the childbirth experience, 'I want to be a midwife to help change the way babies are born' (Van Gorder 2000). Another reason for accepting the spiritual call was the midwife's own belief in, need for, and connection to spirituality: 'reach up to the sky, unite with the source' (Donahue 2000). With each birth, the midwife was aware that she was connected to her universal spiritual source: 'to touch the face of God in the only way I know how while bound to this earth' (Laminack 2000).

When a midwife accepted her calling, she knew that it would be mentally and physically taxing and would require vast amounts of personal investment and energy:

> When it was over, I would pack up with my helpers,
> Go for breakfast. I needed potatoes and bread
> Something of the earth and solid ground,
> Something to remind me of just who I was really,
> Untitled, unknown, a worker – in-service.
>
> (Brendsel 2000b)

One of the primary reasons that being with a woman during childbirth was so exhausting and such hard work, 'I am tired, I am so tired' (Roberts 2001) was because it required heart work: 'you know in your core how to care… it is this that you give, it is this that you share' (Donahue 2000). Being a midwife was a call from the heart, 'for out of the heart, a midwife emerges' (Roberts 2001), and a passion for midwifery that arose from an inner source 'there was this need, or this ache or this something that pushed us forward' (Laminack 2000). In order to fulfil her purpose, the midwife accepted the inherent unpredictability and difficulties of her profession:

The calling that causes us to leave home,
and hearth, and family and friends, and
many denounce comfortable livelihoods...

(Laminack 2000)

She did not become a midwife 'for power, for wealth or for fame'
(Laminack 2000). Instead, the midwife's reward was a spiritual renewal
and connection, 'the smell, the incredible smell of birth, something
that reminds me there is always spring' (Brendsel 2000b), and the realization that by 'being with woman' she had safeguarded another birth
experience:

To be able in the end, to fill the need, soothe
The ache, and live on purpose.
For, I myself, would rather be at a birth
Than to eat or sleep.

(Laminack 2000)

Historical connections

Midwifery was an ancient profession; 'this work is as old as the salt in our
blood' (Whitson 2000). There was a historical essence of spiritual sources
from midwives in the past 'their spirits stand by us in the birth room'
(Whitson 2000) that worked through midwives in the present 'lending their
skills, power and courage to the work of our hands' (Whitson 2000). The
historicity arose from the fact that, as a profession, midwives had always
been by women's sides during labour and birth since the beginning of time:
'women have always birthed with women' (Van Gorder 2000). Midwives
were very aware of and took pride in the fact that their profession had a
lengthy history of 'being with woman':

This work we have done all the length of history
We were there in every place, in every language
Doing this work back through all the days and nights and
Centuries of history
And then further back.

(Whitson 2000)

With this historical knowing of midwifery, 'our souls remember' (Whitson
2000), also came the understanding that birth was a normal process, 'I was
coming out all by myself' (Van Gorder 2000), with no active assistance such
as forceps, and that women knew how to birth, 'I remember well how you
came sliding out wet into the blanket of our arms' (Perdomo 2000d).

Life source connections

The poets used the poems to describe how the midwife knew that there was a part of labour and birth that was controlled by forces other than her own… 'too soon it was for you to come. You were not expected until the first peonies and roses bloomed' (Brendsel 2000a). The midwife also believed that a spiritual source worked through her and guided her safely in her work. She was not afraid of her need for a spiritual relationship as part of her midwifery work, 'oh God I learned to pray' (Brendsel 2000b), and felt in harmony with a belief in spirituality and childbirth:

> the awesome and extreme connection
> Between woman & child
> & the work of birth, the unrelenting spirit
> that charges each to enter
> the ancient caverns of wisdom
> & faith.
>
> (Perdomo 2000a)

After a successful birth experience, the midwife thanked her spiritual source for guidance, 'a prayer of gratitude' (Bowen 2000a) and for substantiating and renewing her worldview that birth was a normal process:

> A prayer of renewal,
> A prayer of life everlasting
> Life, Love and Hope restored.
>
> (Bowen 2000a)

Though 'being with woman' was almost always rewarding and usually ended in a wonderful miraculous birth, 'the welcome wail which signalled life' (Bowen 2000a), there was always the possibility of a complication or even death, 'you rest so still, to small & pale…never troubled by the cares & pains of this world' (Perdomo 2000a). It was this inescapable dimension of childbirth that caused the midwife to ask for spiritual assistance, 'we call you, we invoke your soul in the name of almighty God & holy Trinity' (Perdomo 2000a), in an effort to seek help for those things she could not control and to ask for guidance from her spiritual source: 'a prayer for wisdom, a prayer for guidance' (Bowen 2000a). If the outcome of the complicated birth was successful:

> & then
> slowly so very slowly
> the spirit
> blossoms.
>
> (Perdomo 2000a)

The midwife knew that this was in part because of assistance from a higher spiritual source:

> Vested in mystery
> In things unseen but known,
> Unheard, but known
> untouched, yet sensed…
> you cried.

(Brendsel 2000a)

Partners in birth

The poets believed that in order for the midwife to truly 'be with woman' during labour and childbirth a trusting, reciprocal relationship between midwife and woman was required. The midwife had learned from her informed knowledge that a shared relationship was important to women; 'we will do this together' (Roberts 2001). Through grounded knowledge of lived experience, the midwife knew that when she truly participated in the relationship, 'loving, sharing, caring' (Walsh 1993), the birth experience was more satisfying for the mother, family, and herself. The midwife's self-knowledge that each woman's labour and birth was unique and her very own special experience – 'there is no routine birth' (Walsh 1993) – helped to form a successful partnership with a woman during childbirth. Interpretation of the poetry revealed two sub-themes: (a) birth is a special experience; and (b) partnering.

Birth is a special experience

The poet believed she must treat each woman as an individual, 'this woman' (Whitson 2000), and each birth, 'this birth' (Whitson 2000), as a unique experience. The midwife had to truly 'be with woman' and be part of the relationship, working 'with her' (Whitson 2000) to participate in the uniqueness of the experience. The midwife understood that for the mother and the family members present, each birth was a special experience that could never be replicated. While 'being with woman', the midwife saw how a father was 'steadying the birthwork' (Perdomo 2000d), and how a sister's eyes 'glisten like jewels' (Perdomo 2000d), as she began to understand 'the work of birth' (Perdomo 2000d). The midwife understood that the soon to be born baby would be:

> surrounded by those who
> waited on you
> celebrated by those who
> already loved you.

(Perdomo 2000d)

The midwife knew each birth was special: 'my heart swells… for the miracle of you' (Perdomo 2000a), as she remembered a mother that had marvelled as she 'worked, strained, pushed that infant into the world' (Walsh 1993) or heard a mother whisper, 'I will always remember, your day, our day' (Perdomo 2000d).

She knew that attending a woman during childbirth was not a 'routine delivery…one further procedure in a busy day' (Walsh 1993) but that instead, each birth 'was worth more than blood and riches & …is wealth to us all' (Perdomo 2000c). It was truly an extraordinary occurrence, a miracle, that no single birth was the same:

Sighs,   How hard you were
Sounds little   in coming through the
By little from rising lungs   narrow place of birth
And then you are home   you came to us finally pink
Softly yet.   and breathing.
             (Perdomo 2000a)   (Perdomo 2000c)

The midwife did not view a woman's birth as a 'normal spontaneous delivery' (Walsh 1993) but instead remembered how while she was 'being with woman' she took:

the time
to pause in awe and wonder
as that little head came slowly, ever so slowly,
and the eyes opened and looked out with such trust
and wisdom.

                                                        (Walsh 1993)

Partnering

Partnering was reciprocal co-participation between the midwife and the woman and her family during childbirth. The partnership consisted of a shared venture, the childbirth process, and was an intimate relationship, 'entangled in the limbs and prayer and purpose of another one's hope and body' (Perdomo 2000b), that occurred during a finite frame of time. During the partnership the midwife and the woman worked together as a team, to achieve the common goal of a safe, satisfying birth that was emotionally rewarding. The midwife was a willing partner because of her self-knowledge and beliefs about the following: the purpose of a midwife was 'being with woman is truly being a midwife' (Walsh 1993), birth was a blessed event, 'a sacred mystery' (Perdomo 2000b), women were powerful in birth, 'pulling with the power of labor' (Wildermouth 2000), birth was a normal phenomenon, she 'moans, she cries, tears slip past her eyes, she glows, she rests' (Wildermouth 2000), and women had a right to participate in their own birth with shared decision making 'together we deliver this ONE to life' (Wildermouth 2000). The woman in labour was a willing and important partner in the relationship because it was her pregnancy, her family, her birth and her infant, 'this is how you came to be, mother' (Brendsel 2000a).

Though the relationship during childbirth was usually of a short duration, it consisted of qualities such as intimacy, and trust that are normally experienced in long-term partnerships:

> instantly intimate
> so that breath
> & sweat & the simultaneous
> heart felt moan
> are a common cup grasped
> & shared intensely.
>
> (Perdomo 2000b)

The relationship was intimate and trusted for several reasons. During childbirth, a woman was physically and emotionally vulnerable. Parts of the body that were considered private were often exposed, 'she brings her knees back... forces a disc of dark hair to appear' (Wildermouth 2000). Women expressed psychological vulnerability through intense displays of emotions from pain: 'this hurts so much' (Wildermouth 2000), fear: 'I am frightened' (Roberts 2001), and joy: 'my child, you are here' (Wildermouth 2000). Typically, these were emotions expressed only in the presence of someone with whom one has had a familiar, personal, and intimate relationship.

The poets had a very intimate understanding about the birth process, through all three types of midwifery knowledge (see Figure 10.1 on page 175). The midwife understood the experience of the labouring woman: 'the heart beat of this very earth is pulsing deep in you' (Kalman 2000), and responded by 'being with woman, I respond, I am present' (Roberts 2001). Because of that knowledge, 'I understand what women need from me' (Roberts 2001), midwives were partnered with women and shared the experience of birth using long-term relationship qualities, 'issued to enter the close and private kingdom of marriage and birth' (Perdomo 2000b), on a short term basis: 'it is a license made temporary' (Perdomo 2000b). Part of the shared aspect of partnering with the woman during childbirth was that the midwife was actually present, 'being at the woman's side' (Whitson 2000), and shared in the experience, 'working with her' (Whitson 2000), in whatever capacity the woman desired. Regardless of the type of emotional or physical work required by the midwife, 'my job' (Brendsel 2000b), the midwife was there:

> I am present... I will
> Breath with you, Sigh with you
> Stay up all night with you
> Hold your hands and cry
> Pace the floors with you
> Labor with you.
>
> (Roberts 2001)

Through 'being with woman', the midwife guided the woman and her family members through the childbirth process, 'your new one has arrived' (Kalman 2000), however, she eventually withdrew from the intimate part of the relationship, 'at works ending she will tiptoe away gracefully & unassuming' (Perdomo 2000b). The midwife divested herself from the partnership so that the mother could concentrate on the new long-term intimate relationship she was building with her newborn, 'with the heartbond sealed at first comforting' (Perdomo 2000d). The midwife knew that the mother's relationship with her newborn would become her most important priority, in order to ensure the survival and growth of her child, 'for we are all still children who need loving touch' (Parker 2000), and much more: 'a belly means a family, a culture, a community' (Parker 2000). Because the midwife 'understood Life's plan, Love's touch' (Parker 2000), she was always very careful to end the partnership in an appropriate manner, 'slowly deliberately, you were unswaddled, placed between your mother's breasts' (Brendsel 2000a).

The midwife knew that in the end 'babies go to their mothers' (Brendsel 2000b) and that the midwife went '...back to her own border when the birthwork is done' (Perdomo 2000b). Through the poetic voices of midwives 'being with woman: This is how it was remembered' (Brendsel 2000a).

Findings and the literature

Experienced guidance

Reference to being a guide, and to providing support and guidance as a central component of 'being with woman' is frequently cited in midwifery literature and in qualitative studies of women's experiences of care with a midwife (for example Halldorsdottir and Karlsdottir 1996, Lundgren 2005, Fahy and Parratt 2006, Sjoblom *et al.* 2006, Bayes *et al.* 2008, Lundgren *et al.* 2009). A caring midwife empowered the woman to give birth on her own terms as she guided her through labour. Fahy and Parratt (2006) describe midwifery guardianship as the process of allowing a woman to have an undisturbed birth and to ensure that the midwife and the woman shared power. Part of guardianship included protecting the woman from those who might 'overpower' her and making a safe place for birth. Experienced guidance entailed 'clue reading': knowing when to act, the work of assisting or providing advisement as needed, and when to 'wait watchfully', as one accompanied the woman through the journey of childbirth.

Women felt safe because of their relationship with and trust in the midwife who had knowledge and skills about childbirth (Mander and Melender 2009, Pembroke and Pembroke 2008). Bayes *et al.* (2008), Parratt and Fahy (2008) and Smythe (2003; also refer to Chapter 3) concluded that safety is an abstract and unmeasurable concept. Safe versus unsafe is a terrain that contains the contextual circumstances, honours the particular needs of a woman, and realizes the inherent possibility of childbirth danger. Bayes *et al.* (2008) and Sjoblom *et al.* (2006) report that, in their studies, women felt secure during childbirth because the midwife was competent, attentive, supportive, respectful and accessible, without being in charge of the birth. Fahy and Parratt (2006) discussed the importance of the 'sanctum' as a safe environment that enhanced a woman's embodied power and sense of self.

Qualitative studies pay attention to the voice of women, and to the belief of the midwives in the embodied power arising from successful birth (Lundgren 2005, Sjoblom *et al.* 2006, Bayes *et al.* 2008, John 2009, Mander and Melender 2009). Callister and Freeborn (2007) state that a midwife uses her 'gut feeling' and intuition as a type of experienced knowledge to guide while 'being with woman'. Smythe (2003) explained clinical knowledge as careful listening to yourself, anticipating, waiting, and watching. John's study (2009) describes women giving subtle emotional clues to indicate the amount and type of care and interaction with the midwife they desired. Midwives observed subtle changes in body language and attitude to decide how much guidance they provided. In the work undertaken by Sjoblom *et al.* (2006), women described being allowed their personal space by the midwife as she waited for 'signs' to become involved (Sjoblom *et al.* 2006).

Spiritual connections

Burkhardt (1998) argues that, through the desire of midwives to bring love and healing into the client relationship, we express our spirituality through our intentional presence and by having a conscious desire to be with another. She claimed that this is a conscious interaction of intentionally being present (emotionally, spiritually, physically, and cognitively) in a manner that lets the client feel safe and whole in a sacred space. The most frequent resonance in existing published literature with all three spiritual connection sub-themes was in anecdotal sources and in personal midwifery narratives. Hall (2001) stated that storytelling might be a part of women's spirituality, since it was a way of communicating a sense of self. A further historical and pre-ordained connection for midwifery was the idea that the midwife was the wise woman and conduit for the numerous female goddesses that presided at childbirth in ancient cultures (Rabuzzi 1994).

The midwife understood some forces were uncontrollable during her attendance at childbirth and believed that at times this life source worked through her in her own work. She could ask for spiritual help, with the most common ritual being prayer for assistance. As found in this poetry data set, Chester (1998) described prayer, faith, and spirituality as one of the common threads in 27 personal American midwife narratives. Pembroke and Pembroke (2008) believe that 'being with woman' required a spiritual strength in order to maintain and nurture the intense relationship required during childbirth. Parratt and Fahy (2008) claim that 'being with woman' allowed the midwife to access a non-rational power; an inner source of power and knowing that encompassed her soul and spirit.

Partners in birth

The personal quality of the relationship between women and midwife during childbirth, and the need for it to be genuine, respectful, energized, unique and individualized care is recognized as important by a range of authors (Pembroke and Pembroke 2008, Lundgren *et al.* 2009; also refer to Chapters 5, 7, 8, 9 and 12 for further discussions on the importance of the relationship between mothers and health professionals). Larkin *et al.*'s (2009) concept analysis of women's childbirth experiences found the words 'unique' and 'special' used to describe individual birth experiences. Bayes *et al.* (2008) stated that a positive, reciprocal relationship with the midwife made women feel safe and empowered. The work undertaken by Doherty (2009) on the therapeutic value/alliance in the women-centred midwife–client relationship indicates that collaboration, trust, respect, communication, compassion, presence, empowerment, commitment and the desire to be authentic were important components. Midwives too, valued experiences where they felt like they made a 'special difference' through a reciprocal and caring relationship during a childbirth encounter (Thomas 2006, Hunter *et al.* 2008).

One aspect infrequently discussed, but found in the poetry data was the midwife's skill and importance in starting the new relationship between mother and baby (Kennedy 2000, Lundgren *et al.* 2009).

Methodological strengths and limitations

A strength of this study was the fact that the phenomenological, hermeneutical and Gadamerian philosophical perspective under which the study was conducted was congruent with the type of human science research method van Manen (1997) espoused. The nature of the enquiry, interpretation through writing and reflection, and the use of poetry as data were consistent with phenomenological methodology. In other words I was meticulous about ensuring a correct fit for all components of the study, thereby increasing its credibility and dependability. Sandelowski (2000) stated '...internal coherence within a work is often more important than consensus among scholars or critics of that work' (p. 207).

The varied sample of poetry is a unique form of data for phenomenological examination. Poetry, as data, enhanced the meaning of qualitative work through its textual representation. The segments of poetry that were interwoven throughout the analysis were a strength as they added to the aesthetic value of the interpretations. Indeed, Morse (1995) described connoisseurship (aesthetics) in qualitative research much like that of tasting wine, where one learned to appreciate a particular work for its beauty, originality, and individual substance.

The findings were authenticated by three experienced midwives. Their comments indicated that I had provided a credible interpretation of the data. Van Manen (1997) called the use of a content expert, collaborative assistance, and believed that it strengthened my work.

A limitation to this study is that the poetic data presented a very personalized and idealized version of the midwife and of midwifery, which would not be recognized by many midwives working in many settings across the world. It is clear that these findings can only be transferred to midwives working in similar settings and conditions to those of the midwife poets.

Conclusion

'Being with woman' is a well-established concept of midwifery care that has been further elucidated by the findings of this study. In the poems written by American midwives that form the centre of this chapter, 'being with woman' during childbirth was contextually situated in the relationship between the midwife, the woman and her particular and unique birth experience. Based on the current research it is time to synthesize the findings of studies that have examined 'being with woman' and seek a common, universal language. It is time to move forward as a profession and solicit policy and institutional changes in numerous countries, so midwives can legitimately 'be with woman', and women can be recipients of this normative care.

Browne and Chandra (2009) describe the difficulty in the modern postindustrial society of slowing down enough to truly 'be with woman'. They argue that our fast-paced society does not value this approach or honour the tapestry of individual birth. A midwife cannot easily perform watchful waiting if the institution encourages doing, counting, timing, and charting. Midwives need to continue to challenge unnecessary interventions concerning childbirth, and be steadfast advocates for women/family-centred care. If midwives can 'be with woman' they can 'mark time' by watching, 'take one's time' by acting without hurry, and guard the unique and special 'metrical tempo of time' of each woman during childbirth.

190   *Lauren P. Hunter*

References

American College of Nurse-Midwives (2004) *Philosophy of the American College of Nurse-Midwives.* ACNM: Washington DC.

Bayes S., Fenwick J. and Hauck Y. (2008) A Qualitative analysis of women's short accounts of labour and birth in a Western Australian public Tertiary Hospital. *Journal of Midwifery and Women's Health* 53, 53–61.

Berg M. (2005) A midwifery model of care for childbearing women at high risk: Genuine caring in the caring for the genuine. *Journal of Perinatal Education* 14, 9–21.

Bowen S. (2000a) A midwife's prayer. In: *BirthWork* (ed. L.P. Hunter), 5–6. Pacifica Press: La Jolla.

Bowen S. (2000b) With woman. In: *BirthWork* (ed. L.P. Hunter), 5–6. Pacifica Press: La Jolla.

Brendsel C. (2000a) The gift of the hummingbird. In: *BirthWork* (ed. L.P. Hunter), 7, 9. Pacifica Press: La Jolla.

Brendsel C.(2000b) Sheathed. In: *BirthWork* (ed. L.P. Hunter), 7, 9. Pacifica Press: La Jolla.

Browne J. and Chandra A. (2009) Slow midwifery. *Women and Birth* 22, 29–33.

Burkhardt M. (1998) Reintegrating spirituality into healthcare. *Alternative Therapies in Health and Medicine* 4, 127–128.

Callister L. and Freeborn D. (2007) Nurse midwives with women: Ways of knowing in nurse midwives. *International Journal of Caring* 11, 9–15.

Chester P. (1998) *Sisters on a Journey: Portraits of American Midwives.* Rutgers University Press: Brunswick, NJ.

Cragin L. (2004) The theoretical basis for nurse-midwifery practice in the United States: A critical analysis of three theories. *Journal of Midwifery and Women's Health* 49, 381–389.

Dilthey W. (1987) *Introduction to the Human Sciences.* Scholarly Book Services: Toronto.

Doherty M. (2009) Therapeutic Alliance: A concept for the childbearing season. *The Journal of Perinatal Education* 18, 39–47.

Donahue M. (2000) Caring. In: *BirthWork* (ed. L.P. Hunter), 18. Pacifica Press: La Jolla.

Draper P. (1996) Nursing research and the philosophy of hermeneutics. *Nursing Inquiry* 3, 45–52.

Fahy K. and Parratt A. (2006) Birth territory: A theory for midwifery practice. *Women and Birth* 19, 45–50.

Gadamer H. (1989) *Truth and Method* (2nd rev. edn). (Trans. J. Weinsheimer and D.G. Marshall) Crossroad: New York.

Hall J. (2001) *Midwifery, Mind and Spirit: Emerging Issues of Care.* Books for Midwives: Oxford.

Halldorsdottir S. and Karlsdottir S. (1996) Empowerment or discouragement: Women's experience of caring and uncaring encounters during childbirth. *Health Care Women International* 17, 361–79.

Hunter B., Berg M., Lundgren I., Olafdottir O. and Kirkham M. (2008) Relationships: the hidden threads in the tapestry of maternity care. *Midwifery* 24, 132–137.

Hunter L.P. (2000) *BirthWork.* Pacifica Press: La Jolla.

Hunter L.P. (2002a) Poetry as an aesthetic expression for nursing: a review. *Journal of Advanced Nursing* 40, 141–148.

Hunter L.P. (2002b) Being with Woman: A Guiding concept for the care of laboring women. *Journal of Obstetrical, Gynecological and Neonatal Nursing* 31, 650–657.

Hunter L.P. (2003) An interpretive exploration of the meaning of being with women during birth for midwives. Dissertation: University of San Diego, San Diego.

Hunter L.P. (2008) A hermeneutic phenomenological analysis of midwives' ways of knowing during childbirth. *Midwifery* 24, 405–415.

John V. (2009) A labour of love?: Mothers and emotion work. *British Journal of Midwifery* 17, 636–640.

Kalman J. (2000) Labor song. In: *BirthWork* (ed. L.P. Hunter), 31. Pacifica Press: La Jolla.

Kennedy H. (2000) A model of exemplary midwifery practice: Results of a Delphi study. *Journal of Midwifery and Women's Health* 45, 4–19.

Laminack S. (2000) The calling. In: *BirthWork* (ed. L.P. Hunter), 32. Pacifica Press: La Jolla.

Larkin R., Begley C. and Devane D. (2009) Women's experiences of labour and birth: An evolutionary concept analysis. *Midwifery* 25, 49–59.

Lundgren I. (2005) Swedish women's experiences of childbirth 2 years after birth. *Midwifery* 21, 346–354.

Lundgren I., Karlsdottir S. and Bondas T. (2009) Long term memories and experiences of childbirth in a Nordic context – a secondary analysis. *International Journal of Qualitative Studies on Health and Well-Being* 4, 115–128.

Mander R. and Melender H. (2009) Choice in maternity: Rhetoric, reality and resistance. *Midwifery* 25, 637–648.

Morse G. (1995) Reframing women's health education: A feminist approach. *Nursing Outlook* 43, 273–277.

Parker, K. (2000) In the palm of her hand. *BirthWork* (ed. L.P. Hunter), 41. Pacifica Press: La Jolla.

Parratt J. and Fahy K. (2008) Including the *non*rational is sensible midwifery. *Women and Birth* 21, 37–42.

Pembroke N. and Pembroke J. (2008) The spirituality of presence in midwifery care. *Midwifery* 24, 321–327.

Perdomo E. (2000a) To the doors of heaven. In: *BirthWork* (ed. L.P. Hunter), 43. Pacifica Press: La Jolla.

Perdomo E. (2000b) Birthwork. In: *BirthWork* (ed. L.P. Hunter), 46. Pacifica Press: La Jolla.

Perdomo E. (2000c) Rosie. In: *BirthWork* (ed. L.P. Hunter), 44. Pacifica Press: La Jolla.

Perdomo E. (2000d) Cristina elena. In: *BirthWork* (ed. L.P. Hunter), 43. Pacifica Press: La Jolla.

Rabuzzi K. (1994) *Mother with Child.* University Press: Bloomington, IN.

Roberts S. (2001) Soul work. Unpublished poem. Used with permission.

Sandelowski M. (2000) *Devices and Desires. Gender, Technology and American Nursing.* University of North Carolina Press: Chapel Hill.

Sjoblom I., Nordstrom B. and Edberg A. (2006) A qualitative study of women's experiences of home birth in Sweden. *Midwifery* 22, 348–355.

Smythe E. (2003) Uncovering the meaning of 'being safe' in practice. *Contemporary Nurse* 14, 196–204.

Thomas G. (2006) Making a difference: midwives' experiences of caring for women. *The Royal College of Midwives. Evidence Based Midwifery* 4, 83–88.

Trout A. (2000) A midwife's hands. In: *BirthWork* (ed. L.P. Hunter), 52. Pacifica Press: La Jolla.

VanGorder K. (2000) Remembering. In: *BirthWork* (ed. L.P. Hunter), 53. Pacifica Press: La Jolla.

van Manen M. (1997) *Researching Lived Experience. Human Science for an Action Sensitive Pedagogy.* The Althouse Press: Ontario.

Waldestrom U., Hildingsson I., Rubertsson C. and Radestad I. (2004) A negative birth experience: Prevalence and risk factors in a National Sample. *Birth* 31,17–27.

Walsh L. (1993) The essence of midwifery. In: *On Nursing: A Literary Celebration. An Anthology.* (eds Styles M. and Moccia, P.), 198–200. National League for Nursing: New York.

Whitson N. (2000) Blessing of the hands. In: *BirthWork* (ed. L.P. Hunter), 56. Pacifica Press: La Jolla.

Wildermouth D. (2000) Birth, past, present, future. In: *BirthWork* (ed. L.P. Hunter), 57–58. Pacifica Press: La Jolla.

11 Revealing the subtle differences among postpartum mood and anxiety disorders

Phenomenology holds the key

Cheryl Tatano Beck

Introduction

This chapter begins by presenting the background to the research problem that describes the lack of clarity in differentiating postpartum depression from other mood and anxiety disorders following childbirth. A discussion of the descriptive phenomenological approach undertaken in each of the following three studies is addressed: postpartum depression (Beck 1992), postpartum onset of panic disorder (Beck 1998a), and posttraumatic stress disorder (PTSD) following childbirth (Beck 2004). Details of the samples, data collection, procedures, data analyses and ethical issues involved in these studies are then presented. Results are described and compared and the subtle differences between these postpartum psychiatric disorders are revealed. The methodological challenges faced in conducting these studies are then addressed followed by implications of these phenomenological studies.

Background

The postpartum period is the time in a woman's life when she is most vulnerable to developing psychiatric disorders. There is an array of postpartum mood and anxiety disorders that can strike new mothers. Postpartum mood disorders include postpartum depression, bipolar II disorders – called the postpartum depression imposter (Beck and Driscoll 2006), and postpartum psychosis. Postpartum anxiety disorders include panic disorder with postpartum onset, obsessive compulsive disorder with postpartum onset, and posttraumatic stress disorder (PTSD) due to birth trauma.

In the Agency for Healthcare Research and Quality (AHRQ) evidence report the prevalence of major and minor depression at three months postpartum was 19.2 per cent (Gavin *et al.* 2005). Of the limited number of studies examining the prevalence of postpartum onset of panic disorder, Reck *et al.* (2008) reported a prevalence rate of 1.8 per cent in their sample of 1,024 postpartum women; while Matthey *et al.* (2003) identified a rate of 2.7 per cent in their sample of 408 women six weeks after birth. In a US national survey, 'Listening to Mothers II Postpartum Survey', 8.9 per cent of mothers screened positive for meeting the diagnostic criteria for PTSD due to childbirth (Declercq *et al.* 2008).

Clinical presentation of postpartum anxiety disorders has received much less research attention than postpartum depression (Ross and McLean 2006). The full spectrum of postpartum psychiatric disorders is poorly understood and therefore can be either misdiagnosed or under diagnosed (Halbreich 2005). The consequences of misdiagnosis are especially critical in the postpartum period because of the detrimental effect that inappropriate treatment can have on mother–infant bonding (Sharma *et al.* 2008).

Bernstein *et al.* (2008) noted that there has been a paucity of research concentrating on symptoms unique to women after birth. Despite compelling evidence that postpartum psychiatric disorders are not limited to depression, Marrs *et al.* (2009) reported that there are few studies that have been conducted on specific symptoms in postpartum women. The differentiation between postpartum depression and other types of depression is often unclear (Craig and Howard 2009).

Sharma (2002) has suggested that research studies comparing symptom patterns in mothers with major depression and bipolar depression during the postpartum period are urgently needed, as are strategies to decrease misdiagnosis of subtle forms of postpartum mood and anxiety disorders. The correct diagnosis is critical to minimizing potential adverse consequences to mothers and their infants. Sharma *et al.* (2008) examined the diagnostic profile and co-morbidity patterns of 56 women referred for follow up with a diagnosis of postpartum depression. Fifty-four per cent of women with postpartum depression had a bipolar spectrum disorder. These authors called for phenomenological studies to compare postpartum mood and anxiety disorders to help prevent misdiagnosis.

The results of three phenomenological studies undertaken by the author to explore women's experiences of postnatal depression (Beck 1992); postpartum onset of panic disorder (Beck 1998a) and posttraumatic stress disorder following childbirth (Beck 2004) are now presented. This is followed by a synthesis of the findings to illuminate how phenomenological insights can reveal the subtle differences between postpartum mood and anxiety disorders.

Methodology

Theoretical perspective

A descriptive phenomenological approach was used in all three studies (an overview of all the three studies presented in this chapter is shown in Table 11.1). The aim of descriptive phenomenology is to describe the meaning of human experience as it is viewed by persons who have had that experience (also discussed in Chapters 1 and 4). The intention is to describe what makes a phenomenon what it is and without which it could not be what

Table 11.1 Comparison of methodology of three descriptive phenomenological studies of postpartum mood and anxiety disorders

	Postpartum depression	*Postpartum panic disorder*	*Posttraumatic stress disorder (PTSD) due to childbirth*
Research question	'What is the lived experience of postpartum depression?'	'What is the essential structure of experiences of panic in mothers who developed onset of panic disorder after delivery?'	'What is the essence of mothers' experiences of PTSD after traumatic births?'
Data analysis	Colaizzi (1973, 1978)	Colaizzi (1973, 1978)	Colaizzi (1973, 1978)
Data collection	In-person interviews	In-person interviews	Internet interviews
Sample size	7 women	6 women	38 women
Interview statement	'Please describe a situation in which you experienced postpartum depression.'	'Please describe your experiences living with panic disorder during the postpartum period.'	'Please describe your experiences of PTSD after childbirth.'
Results	11 themes: • Unbearable loneliness • Suicidal thoughts • Obsessive thinking • Loss of self • Lack of previous interests • Suffocating guilt • Cognitive impairment • Devoid of positive feelings • Uncontrollable anxiety • Loss of control • Besieged with insecurities	6 themes: • Terrifying physical and emotional components of panic attacks • Diminished cognitive functioning • Struggling to keep panic attacks down • Preventing panic attacks became paramount • Lowered self-esteem due to changes in women's lifestyles • Haunted by the fear that their panic attacks could have residual effects	5 themes: • Going to the movies: 'Please don't make me go' • A shadow of myself: 'Too numb to try and change' • Seeking answers • A dangerous trio of anger, anxiety and depression • Isolation from the world of motherhood

it is (Husserl 1913). One assumption of descriptive phenomenology is that for any human experience there are distinct essential structures that comprise that experience regardless of the specific person who experiences it. The phenomenon being studied needs to be described as it is consciously experienced without any theories about its cause and as free as possible of any unexamined presuppositions of the researcher (Spiegelberg 1975). Husserl (1960) called for the process of phenomenologic reduction in order for these essential structures to be understood. In reduction, researchers attempt to 'bracket' or hold aside and suspend temporarily their preconceptions about the phenomenon under study in order to allow this phenomenon to come directly into view and not be distorted by the researchers' presuppositions. Husserl called for complete reduction; however, other philosophers, such as Merleau-Ponty (1956) argued that 'the greatest lesson of reduction is the impossibility of a complete reduction' (p. 64).

Study one: Postpartum depression

Sample method

A purposive sample of seven women participated in the study (Beck 1992). The age range of the mothers was 22 to 38. Four women were primiparas and three were multiparas. Three women had caesarean births, while four had vaginal births. Six of the seven mothers were under the care of a psychiatrist for their postpartum depression. All the women were married and Caucasian.

Recruitment method

Women were recruited in the southeastern United States from a local postpartum depression support group which the researcher helped to facilitate.

Procedure/data collection

After the study received Institutional Review Board approval from the researcher's university, women were approached to participate in the study. Once informed consent was obtained women were asked to respond verbally to the following statement: 'Please describe a situation in which you experienced postpartum depression. Share all the thoughts, perceptions and feelings you can recall until you have no more to say about the situation' (Beck 1992, p. 167). Women were privately interviewed by the researcher. Interviews were tape recorded and transcribed verbatim.

Ethical issues

If women became upset describing their experiences of postpartum depression, they were told by the researcher that they did not have to finish the interview. There was also a mechanism in place to refer women for follow up with a mental health professional if that was deemed necessary.

Study two: Postpartum onset of panic disorder

Sample method

The purposive sample consisted of six mothers who had been diagnosed with postpartum onset of panic disorder (Beck 1998a). Five women were multiparas and one was a primipara. All the women were married. Five women were Caucasian and one mother was born in Cambodia.

Recruitment method

Women were referred to the researcher in three ways: (1) by a nurse psychotherapist in private practice; (2) by a nurse who had previously been a leader of a postpartum depression support group; and (3) by two women who were co-leaders of a local chapter of Depression after Delivery.

Procedure/data collection

After receiving approval from the university's Institutional Review Board, women were referred to the researcher. Once informed consent was signed, each woman was privately interviewed by the researcher. All interviews were tape recorded and transcribed verbatim. Each woman was asked to describe her experiences living with panic during her post-partum period. The length of the interviews ranged from 50 minutes to two hours.

Ethical issues

If women became upset describing their experiences of postpartum onset of panic disorder, they were told by the researcher that they did not have to finish the interview. There was also a mechanism in place to refer women for follow up with a mental health professional if that was needed.

Study three: Posttraumatic stress disorder due to childbirth

Sample method

The convenience sample included 38 women representing four countries. Twenty-two women were from New Zealand, seven women from the United States, six mothers from Australia, and three mothers from the United Kingdom. The mean age of the sample was 33 years. Twenty-six mothers were multiparas and 12 were primiparas. Seventeen women had caesarean births and 21 had vaginal births. Focusing on marital status, 34 women were married, two were single, and two were divorced.

Recruitment method

Women were recruited through the assistance of Trauma and Birth Stress (TABS), a charitable trust located in New Zealand.[1] A recruitment notice for the study was placed in TABS newsletter plus the chairperson of TABS sent a letter to the members of TABS informing them of the study.

Procedure/data collection

Interested women contacted the researcher via her university email address. Directions for the study and an informed consent sheet were then sent on attachment. Participants electronically signed the informed consent and sent it back to the researcher on attachment. Women were asked to write their experiences of PTSD due to birth trauma in as much detail as they wished and could remember. Since this study was conducted via the Internet, women sent their completed stories on attachment to the researcher.

Ethical issues

Because the researcher was not physically present with the women as they participated in the Internet study (Beck 2004), a different approach was used in case women became upset or anxious remembering their traumatic births. Women were told in the informed consent sheet that if they became anxious or upset writing their stories on the computer, they should stop and discuss their feelings with either their therapist or a family member or friend. It was also stressed to the women that they did not need to complete the study even if they had signed the informed consent.

Data analysis in all the studies

Colaizzi's (1973, 1978) method of phenomenological data analysis was used in all three studies. Colaizzi identified four sources of descriptive data in a phenomenological study: written descriptions, dialogical interviews, observation, and imaginative presence. For each data source he has a corresponding data analysis method. Written descriptions were the source of data in the three phenomenological studies presented in this chapter. Protocol analysis is Colaizzi's (1978) data analysis method for written descriptions and so this analysis approach was used in these studies. This consists of seven procedural steps which are illustrated in Figure 11.1.

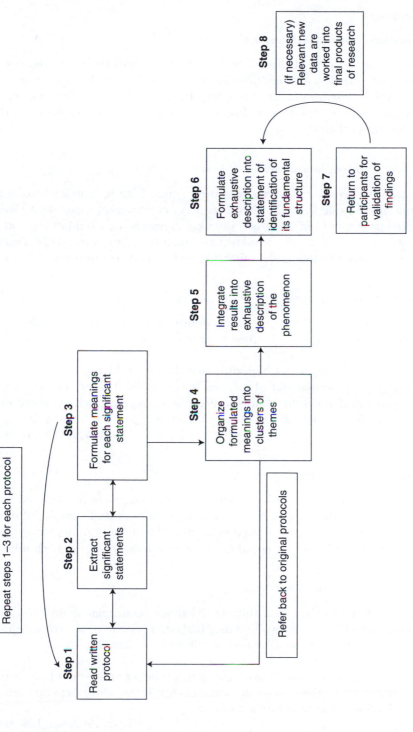

Figure 11.1 Colaizzi's (1973, 1978) procedural steps for analysing data phenomenolgically.
Reprinted with permission from Beck and Watson (2008).

Findings

Study one: Postpartum depression

The seven mothers in this study described in depth their experiences of living with this devastating illness. They shared many detailed, specific examples which were invaluable in helping the themes emerge. The essence of the participants' experiences of postpartum depression was captured by the following 11 themes.

Theme 1: Unbearable loneliness

Women perceived that no one, not their family, friends, nor clinicians, truly understood the depths of the nightmare they were struggling to survive. Mothers would try in vain to explain what they were experiencing but they were told to 'just snap out of it', move on and focus on their beautiful, healthy baby. Due to these unsuccessful attempts, mothers were enveloped in unbearable loneliness.

Theme 2: Suicidal thoughts

As women plunged farther into the depths of postpartum depression, the idea of leaving this world became enticing. It was like:

> going to the gates of hell and back. It was terrifying. I felt there was absolutely no way out of it. I was very suicidal. I loved my baby but I thought if this is the quality of life that I was going to have, there's no way. No way anybody can endure the kind of pain I was going through.
>
> (Beck 1992, p. 168)

Theme 3: Obsessive thinking

Day and night women with postpartum depression were bombarded with obsessive thoughts that kept racing through their minds. Examples of these thoughts that constantly haunted mothers included questioning if they were going crazy, and why they could not love their baby the way they should.

Theme 4: Loss of self

Women were terrified that they would never be normal again; that they would never be the same women they had been prior to postpartum depression. Mothers mourned their loss of self. As Lisa admitted:

> My big fear was that I wasn't going to get better and even if I got better that I wasn't going to be the same person I was before the experience; that I never would quite get over it.
>
> (Beck 1992, pp. 168–169)

Theme 5: Lack of interest in previous activities

Any hobbies, interests or activities that once brought women enjoyment in their lives no longer brought them any solace from their postpartum depression.

Theme 6: Suffocating guilt

Consuming guilt filled mothers. So much guilt to go around; guilt over not giving their infants the love they felt the babies needed; guilt over horrific thoughts of harming their infants; guilt over the possibility of psychologically harming their infants. As Nicole painfully shared:

> I always worried about my son. I knew I couldn't take care of him but I was always asking my mom to hold him and love him for me. I didn't want him to suffer. The guilt made it even worse and the fact I couldn't love him normally made it even worse.
>
> (Beck 1992, p. 169)

Theme 7: Cognitive impairment

Women repeatedly shared that while suffering with postpartum depression their ability to concentrate was diminished. Feeling like fogginess was setting in their brains or their minds were filled with cobwebs were two images that were frequently used to try and explain what they were experiencing.

> If I went grocery shopping, it was like I was in a fog. I would do it but it would take me 4 hours to unload the bags and put them away. It was as if I just wasn't efficient at anything. Everything was a big, big deal to do.
>
> (Beck 1992, p. 169)

Theme 8: Devoid of positive feelings

'Robots just going through the motions' and 'zombies' were two phrases mothers often used to try and capture the enveloping feelings of emptiness they suffered. Anxiety, fear, and sadness were the emotions they felt. No joy or love while caring for their infants was experienced. Positive emotions were longed for, but not to be. Women described themselves as acting and not feeling real as the withdrawal of positive emotions occurred:

> I'd be having guests or family over for dinner and laughing and talking. All of a sudden it was like my personality was pulled right out of me and I'd just be quiet and look around. I'd start acting again.
>
> (Beck 1992, p. 169)

Theme 9: Uncontrollable anxiety

Postpartum depressed women not only suffered with sadness but also with anxiety. For some mothers the anxiety was much worse than the sadness. Women described that they could not keep still but had to keep moving and pacing. The anxiety at times became too intense. Women felt like they were losing their minds. Here is an insider's description of this anxiety:

> It's terrible. It's like the worst thing you can imagine. Think of how you would feel if your husband or child had been hit by a car and killed. Well, it would be as bad as what I felt during an anxiety attack.
>
> (Beck 1992, p. 169)

Theme 10: Loss of control

Loss of control was the basic problem postpartum depressed women had to try and cope with. It permeated all aspects of their lives, their emotions and their thoughts:

> I had no control and that was the scary thing. I felt trapped. I felt like there was absolutely no way out of this hell. These horrible feelings weren't going to leave no matter how hard I tried.
>
> (Beck 1992, p. 169)

Theme 11: Besieged with insecurities

Mothers described themselves as vulnerable, fragile, and weak which left them feeling extremely insecure in their role as a new mother. The responsibilities of motherhood were overwhelming. Women shared that if they could not control their thoughts or emotions, how could they depend on themselves to care for their tiny, helpless infants.

> It just snapped in me and there was no going back. Even though all of a sudden everybody rushed in to help, it didn't make any difference. I was like an infant. I had to be with my mother all the time. I needed help with the baby. The responsibility seemed absolutely enormous.
>
> (Beck 1992, p. 170)

Study two: Postpartum onset of panic disorder

Through the in depth interviews carried out with the six women in this study, a powerful picture emerged as the six themes were fitted together like a puzzle to portray the essential meanings.

Theme 1: Terrifying physical and emotional components of panic attacks

Women felt totally out of control when the terrifying physical and emotional components during panic attacks occurred. Physical symptoms such as chest pain, heart palpitations and shortness of breath resulted in mothers feeling distraught as they tried desperately to 'keep the panic down'. Nancy vividly described her terrifying panic attacks:

> My body always felt hot. I feel hot tears, hot flashes, and most of the time I feel hot inside of my head. I feel shaky. It seemed that every time I closed my eyes, something broke out in my head. It is like the noise, the sound of my computer. I feel pain. It starts from the bottom of my feet up to my head. I feel like the blood is moving up to my head faster and faster. My face is hot. I fear the pain, the muscle spasms over my heart. I start to feel am I going to have a stroke? It is getting worse and worse. It spread. I fear it might damage my heart.
>
> (Beck 1998a, p. 133)

Theme 2: Diminished cognitive functioning

While in the throws of a terrifying panic attack, mothers' cognitive functioning abruptly diminished as women felt like they were losing their minds. Between panic attacks, a more insidious decrease in women's cognitive functioning occurred. Mothers' ability to concentrate was hindered as their fear of the next panic attack distracted and consumed their thoughts. Fearing that her cognitive ability was diminished, Kim started audio taping her child and painfully shared:

> When he is 15, I want to listen to his voice when he was a baby so that I can hear it when I am normal. Because I am not sure now that when I hear him babbling and gooing, that what I am even hearing is normal.
>
> (Beck 1998a, p. 133)

Theme 3: Struggling to keep panic attacks down

During panic attacks women feverishly struggled to keep their composure. So much energy was expended trying to hide the fact from others that they were experiencing a panic attack. Mothers desperately tried to 'keep the panic down' but to no avail. Once a panic attack was over, women reported that exhaustion set in.

Theme 4: Preventing panic attacks became paramount

The excerpt, 'my life was completely consumed with panic prevention which was motivated mainly by my own hyper vigilance to appear "normal" and not to disgrace my family' (Beck 1998a, p. 134) captures what mothers experienced. Because women were so terrified of having another panic attack, they sought to discover what the specific panic triggers were for themselves. Certain times of the day, certain phases of their menstrual cycle, being confined indoors, and being away from their infants were examples of what would trigger panic attacks.

Theme 5: Lowered self-esteem due to changes in women's lifestyles

In their frantic attempts to prevent further panic attacks, women drastically curtailed their regular daily activities. Some women refused to leave the safety of their homes for fear of triggering an onset. Plummeting self-esteem left mothers feeling totally incompetent in their role as a mother. Mothers anguished over their belief that they had repeatedly let their families down because of their panic. The heart-wrenching disappointment some women experienced in themselves as a result of their panic was quite apparent in the passage that follows. Michelle could not bear to attend story hour at the library and said:

> I can't believe I could be so disappointed in myself. I couldn't bear that my son was losing out. I don't know. I guess I really just wanted him to enjoy story hour like all the other kids but when I got home I just cried. I cried for hours 'cause I felt like I was a bad mother. I was just so disappointed in myself but we never went back.
>
> (Beck 1998a, p. 134)

Theme 6: Haunted their panic could have residual effects

Women feared that their recurring panic attacks would traumatize their infants and older children.

> I was so afraid that I would leave a permanent mark on my son. That the way I was would rub off on him. I just wished for his life that he can do well in spite of me somehow.
>
> (Beck 1998a, p. 134)

Mothers also feared that they would never completely recover from the panic attacks. They were vehement in the belief that the terrifying memories of their panic would be imprinted in their minds forever.

Study three: PTSD following childbirth

The 38 mothers who took part in this study provided powerful testimony that resulted in five emergent themes.

Theme 1: Going to the movies – please don't make me go

Flashbacks and nightmares of their traumatic births tormented the women. The image of a video on automatic replay in their brains continually playing their traumatic births was frequently used by the mothers. These loop tracks imprinted in their brains left women 'stuck in the past' preventing them from enjoying motherhood. Meredith, who had a forceps delivery following a failed vacuum extraction, revealed:

> I lived in two worlds, the videotape of the birth and the 'real' world. The videotape felt more real. I lived in my own bubble, not quite connecting with anyone. I could hear and communicate, but experienced interaction with others as a spectator. The 'videotape' ran constantly for 4 months.
>
> (Beck 2004, p. 219)

Deborah, who had an 'agonizing forceps delivery', reported that she was plagued with 'extraordinarily realistic nightmares'. She described that:

> like Lady MacBeth, I became terrified of sleeping! I would go without sleep for about 72 to 96 hours. I always knew I'd have to fight the nightmares again. I was scared that this time I wouldn't have the strength to fight it, that it would succeed in destroying me.
>
> (Beck 2004, p. 219)

Theme 2: A shadow of myself: too numb to try and change

When experiencing PTSD following childbirth, women described themselves as only a shadow of their former selves, feeling numb and detached. 'I'd wake up numb unable to feel a thing. I'd drag myself though the day. I am having the hardest time trying to overcome this feeling of being dead' (Beck 2004, p. 220).

Theme 3: Seeking answers

What had gone so wrong with their dream of giving birth? Mothers who experienced PTSD obsessed over getting answers in an attempt to understand what had happened. Examples of this obsession included revisiting the delivery room, reading obstetrical text books, and surfing the Internet in their search for answers to the questions that haunted them.

Family, friends, and clinicians became tired of listening to their repeated questions and Denise admitted:

> I was so devastated at people's lack of empathy. I told myself what a bad person I was for needing to talk. I felt like the Ancient Mariner doomed

to forever be plucking at people's sleeves and trying to tell them my story which they didn't want to hear.

(Beck 2004, p. 221)

Theme 4: Dangerous trio of anger, anxiety and depression

Mothers struggling with PTSD due to a traumatic childbirth experienced these distressing emotions on a heightened level. Anger turned to rage at times; anxiety led to panic attacks, and as their depression deepened, suicidal thoughts started to creep in their minds. This distressing emotion was vividly described as:

I wanted to kill myself. My life was a mess. Death seemed like a wonderful idea. I'd fight with myself while driving, 'Put your foot on the brake, the light's red. No, don't put your foot on the brake', and so it went on.

(Beck 2004, p. 222)

Louise revealed:

Powerful seething anger would overwhelm me without warning. To manage it I would go still and quiet, then eventually 'come to', realizing that one or all of the children were crying and I had no idea for how long.

(Beck 2004, p. 221)

Theme 5: Isolation from world of motherhood

Any person with PTSD goes to great lengths to avoid triggers of their traumatic event. For women with PTSD due to birth trauma, any reminders of motherhood were triggers: for example their infants and other mothers. This theme has tremendous implications for mother–infant bonding. There were also long term effects of PTSD:

My child turned 3 years old a few weeks ago. I suppose the pain was not so acute this time. I actually made him a birthday cake and was grateful that I could go to work and not think about this significance of the day. The pain was less, but it was replaced by a numbness that still worries me. I hope that as time passes I can forge some kind of real closeness with this child. I am still unable to tell him I love him, but I can now hold him and have times when I am proud of him. I have come a long, long way.

(Beck 2004, p. 222)

Discussion

Subtle differences in symptom patterns

With the help of these three phenomenological studies, subtle differences were discovered that hopefully will help decrease the misdiagnosis of these crippling disorders in new mothers (Beck 1992, 1998a, 2004). Using phenomenology as the research method allowed women's vivid and powerful detailed descriptions of these mood and anxiety disorders to come alive. Nuances in the diagnostic profiles emerged as the researcher was able to 'walk a mile in their shoes.'

Loneliness/isolation

Mothers suffering with all three postpartum disorders experienced loneliness and isolation. However, discrete differences were revealed by the participants. In postpartum depression loneliness prevailed because of the women's belief that no one really understood the depths of their despair. Women tried to explain this to family, friends, and even health care providers but as their pleas for understanding fell on deaf ears, mothers started to isolate themselves due to the discomfort of being around other people.

With postpartum onset of panic disorder women also isolated themselves, however, for a different reason. Fearing the onset of another dreaded panic attack some mothers drastically reduced their daily activities and isolated themselves at home. At least if a panic attack occurred, women would be in the safety of their own homes.

Isolation permeated the lives of women with PTSD due to childbirth. As with postpartum depression, these women also felt that others did not truly understand what they were going through.

> Not only does PTSD isolate me from the outside world; it isolates me even from those I love. How do I explain the sort of blind terror that overtakes me without warning and without obvious logical cause? And what of my family and friends? They don't know how I feel. They don't know what to say, and they cannot make it better, so they end up feeling useless. That's the real problem with PTSD. It separates people at the time when love and understanding are most needed. It's like an invisible wall around the sufferer.
>
> (Beck 2004, p. 221)

This isolation was further compounded by women's avoidance of any triggers of their traumatic births that could lead to terrifying flashbacks. Mothers purposely isolated themselves from reminders of birth: for example other mothers and their infants and their own infants. Caron painfully shared the isolation and heartache she felt due to the invisible walls her birth trauma erected between herself and her infant:

> At night I tried to connect/acknowledge in my heart that this was my son and I cried. I knew that there were great layers of trauma around my heart. I wanted to feel motherhood. I wanted to experience and embrace it. Why was I chained up in the vicelike grip of this pain? This was my Gethsemane – my agony in the garden.
>
> (Beck 2004, p. 222)

Cognitive impairment

Diminished ability to concentrate and make decisions was experienced in all three puerperal psychiatric disorders. Again, however, subtle differences were discovered by the phenomenological studies. Women suffering with postpartum depression described the fog rolling into their brains clouding their cognitive ability. There was not any specific reason why and when this fogginess appeared.

In postpartum onset of panic disorder and PTSD following birth, more specific reasons for this diminished cognitive ability were identified. With postpartum onset of panic disorders women took a double hit on their cognitive ability. First, during the actual panic attacks their cognitive functioning abruptly decreased. Women described their thinking during panic attacks as irrational. They would make catastrophic misinterpretations of the physical symptoms they experienced such as:

> During the panic attacks, I would have chest pains and shortness of breath. I thought I was having a heart attack and I was going to die. I remember having gone to the emergency room a few times just to have someone tell me that I was okay. They said I was abusing the emergency room. It was just for an emergency!
>
> (Beck 1998a, p. 133)

Between panic attacks, mothers' cognitive functioning was still diminished. This was a more chronic problem, however, as the fear of another panic attack distracted mothers as they were consumed with worry.

PTSD following a traumatic childbirth also affected mothers' cognitive functioning. When experiencing the unexpected flashbacks to their birth trauma, cognitive impairment occurred.

Obsessive thoughts

With all three postpartum mood and anxiety disorders, mothers waking hours were often filled with obsessive thoughts. For postpartum depressed mothers this thinking consisted of being bombarded by constant questioning such as, 'What is wrong with me?', 'Am I going crazy?', 'Why can't I love my baby the way I should?'. In postpartum onset of panic disorder, mothers' thoughts were consumed by preventing further panic attacks. It was similar to detective work as women constantly tried to identify what were the triggers that would set off another dreaded attack. With PTSD due to birth trauma, mothers could not control the videotape of their birth trauma in their minds. It was on automatic replay leaving the feeling of loop tracks in their brains.

Loss of control

Mothers described that with postpartum depression they could not control any aspect of their lives; not their emotions nor their thoughts. Molly divulged that, 'I had no control and that was the scary thing. I felt trapped. I felt like there was absolutely no way out of this hell. These horrible feelings weren't going to leave no matter how hard I tried' (Beck 1992, p. 169)

With panic disorder in the postpartum period, women had no control whatsoever regarding when a panic attack would strike. The terrifying physical and emotional components of a panic attack paralysed mothers and left them feeling totally out of control. Women trying to cope with PTSD following childbirth also experienced loss of control but theirs was in relation to the flashbacks and nightmares of the traumatic events.

Women with postpartum depression and PTSD due to birth trauma described loss of control in relation to anger. Irritability and anger were part of the profile of postpartum depressed mothers: 'Many times I would be on the verge of throwing my son at my husband' (Beck 1992, p. 169).

Anger filled a large portion of mothers' lives with PTSD. Their anger lashed out in multiple directions: Anger at the clinicians present during their labour and delivery for betraying her trust, anger at their partners and other support persons in childbirth who did not stand up for them, and anger at themselves for letting the traumatic birth occur.

Loss of self

Participants in all three phenomenological studies mourned the loss of their normal selves and were terrified their lives would never be right again.

Anxiety

Anxiety was a component of the symptom profile in all three of these postpartum mood and anxiety disorders. In postpartum onset of panic disorder, however, this anxiety escalated to panic. During panic attacks mothers shared they would have to endure palpitations, chest pains, sweating, shortness of breath, nausea, dizziness, feeling unreal, fear of dying or going crazy, and hot flushes.

Insecurity

No matter which of these mood and anxiety disorders mothers had, they all experienced being insecure. For women who anguished with postpartum onset of panic disorder, their insecurity came from being on edge dreading when the next panic attack would strike. Whereas with mothers suffering from PTSD, it was the fear of the next flashback to their traumatic child-birth which rendered them insecure.

Guilt

Guilt pervaded mothers' lives with all three of these postpartum mood and anxiety disorders. Important subtle differences in how this guilt was experienced were again able to be illuminated through the phenomenological approach of these studies. In postpartum depression mothers bore the suffocating burden of guilt due to their inability to love their infants the way that should and for their horrific thoughts of harming their infants. Mothers suffering with postpartum onset of panic disorder also bore a heavy burden of guilt. These women's guilt hinged on their belief they had disappointed their infants and families. Mothers' self-esteem plummeted and their guilt skyrocketed as they drastically curtailed their normal, everyday activities. With PTSD following childbirth, women's guilt festered as a consequence of the distance mothers felt their birth trauma had created between themselves and their infants.

Lack of positive emotions

Postpartum depressed women repeatedly spoke of feeling like a robot, devoid of all positive feelings, just going through the motions caring for their infants. Women struggling with PTSD due to birth trauma often shared they felt numb and detached. The negative emotions consuming women with panic disorders included constant fear of the next panic attack, plummeting self-esteem and heart wrenching disappointment in them selves. There was no room left for any positive emotions.

Loss of interest

Yet again women with these psychiatric disorders experienced this symptom profile but subtle differences were apparent. In postpartum depression, mothers' depressed mood deprived women of any enjoyment in any of their previous interests. In panic disorder it was the fear of recurring panic attacks that resulted in negative changes in their life styles. These mothers avoided their previous interests in hope of preventing another panic attack. Mothers suffering with PTSD expressed a general apathy towards anything concerning motherhood. This lack of interest was generally fuelled by attempts to avoid triggers that would initiate yet another terrifying flashback or nightmare.

Suicidal thoughts

No matter which postpartum mood and anxiety disorder mothers were suffering, at times some women did contemplate ending their lives; however, this was mainly reported in mothers suffering with postpartum depression. For these mothers, suicidal thoughts stemmed from the tremendous guilt they felt for being 'such bad mothers'. These women were tormented over not loving their infants as much as they thought they should, or having horrific thoughts of harming their infants.

Reflections on the use of the Internet for phenomenological study

Colaizzi's (1978) existential phenomenological method was used in all three studies of postpartum mood and anxiety disorders. What differed, however, was how the data were collected. In depth, one-on-one interviews were conducted in the studies of postpartum depression and postpartum onset of panic disorder. For the PTSD due to birth trauma study, email interviews were conducted. Prior to the PTSD following traumatic childbirth study, the researcher had always conducted in-person interviews with the mothers in her phenomenological studies. This approach yielded rich description with vivid, powerful examples from the participants. This led to reservations about the quality of the data that could be produced by using an Internet based approach for the PTSD due to birth trauma study, given the lack of opportunity for face-to-face meeting. In the end, the vivid descriptions provided by the mothers via the Internet far exceeded expectations. On reflection, given the sensitive nature of the subject, it is possible that even richer data were produced than might have been obtained through in-person interviews. Participants shared that writing down their experiences of PTSD due to their traumatic childbirths was difficult and at times anxiety provoking and so they needed to take breaks from writing their stories, perhaps for a day or weeks at a time. Typing their stories on the computer made it easy for the women to save their partially completed stories in a file and then call them back up when they felt they were ready to write more about their experiences. During an in-person interview with the researcher there would only have been so much remembering of their PTSD experiences that the mothers could have handled at one sitting.

Strengths and limitations of the research method

Phenomenology as a research method is a perfect fit conceptually with the kinds of research questions that emerge in clinical practice disciplines, such as nursing and psychology. This approach affords clinicians a different way to interpret an individual's involvement in the world. Phenomenological studies allow the readers to have a privileged insider's glimpse of what it is like to experience a phenomenon, such as posttraumatic stress disorder following traumatic childbirth. Clinicians can use these valuable findings to design specific interventions.

Using the Internet as a data collection method in phenomenological studies has both advantages and disadvantages. One strength of Internet samples is that web users are from around the globe so that international samples can be recruited easily. A limitation is that the participants tend to be more highly educated and have higher incomes than non-Internet users. Because of this profile, the transferability of the findings from the PTSD following birth trauma study may be limited.

However, unexpectedly, the Internet participants reported they had reaped the following benefits: felt cared for my being listened to and acknowledged, felt a sense of belonging, felt empowered, helped make sense of their traumatic experiences, helped them let go of these traumatic memories, and provided them a voice (Beck 2005).

Implications for clinical practice

Findings from these three phenomenological studies on postpartum mood and anxiety disorders provide valuable data that both clinicians and researchers can use to improve clinical practice. Comparison of the themes discovered in each study helped to tease out subtle differences that clinicians can use to prevent misdiagnosis of these postpartum mood and anxiety disorders. Qualitative results from phenomenological studies are an invaluable source of items that researchers can use for instrument development. The researcher used the findings from her phenomenological study (Beck 1992) of the lived experience of postpartum depression to develop the Postpartum Depression Checklist (PDC) (Beck 1998b). The PDC was developed as an informal checklist to be used by clinicians in a dialogue with new mothers. It consists of 11 symptoms mothers can suffer with when experiencing postpartum depression. Each of the 11 symptoms was derived from one of the 11 themes from the phenomenological study. The PDC can help health care providers to identify women who might be suffering from postpartum depression and might need to be referred to mental health professionals for follow up.

The best way we can ensure the safety of our children is to ensure the mental health of their mothers. The best way we can promote the mental health of new mothers suffering with a postpartum mood and anxiety disorder is to provide them with a quick, accurate diagnosis. Misdiagnosis leads to a prolonged decrease in the quality of life not only for new mothers but also for their entire families. Use of phenomenology as a research method provided valuable, subtle differences between three postpartum mood and anxiety disorders that clinicians can use to facilitate making correct diagnoses.

Conclusion

In this chapter, the invaluable use of phenomenology in revealing subtle differences in postpartum mood and anxiety disorders was illustrated. The specific mental disorders addressed were postpartum depression, postpartum onset of panic disorder, and PTSD due to childbirth. The theoretical perspective of descriptive phenomenology was discussed along with the methodology used in the three phenomenological studies. The essential themes that emerged from using Colaizzi's data analysis (1978) helped to differentiate postpartum depression from two types of postpartum anxiety disorders. Clinicians can use these findings to help prevent making misdiagnoses of new mothers suffering from these postpartum psychiatric disorders.

Note

1 TABS's aims are to provide support for women who have experienced traumatic childbirth and to educate health care providers and lay public about PTSD due to childbirth (www.tabs.org.nz).

References

Beck C. T. (1992). The lived experience of postpartum depression. A phenomenological study. *Nursing Research* 41, 166–170.

Beck C. T. (1998a). Postpartum onset of panic disorder. *Image: Journal of Nursing Scholarship* 30, 131–135.

Beck C. T. (1998b). Screening methods for postpartum depression. *Journal of Obstetric, Gynecologic, and Neonatal Nursing* 24, 308–312.

Beck C .T. (2004). Post-traumatic stress disorder due to childbirth: The aftermath. *Nursing Research* 53, 216–224.

Beck C. T. (2005). Benefits of participating in Internet interviews: Women helping women. *Qualitative Health Research* 15, 411–422.

Beck C. T. and Driscoll J. W. (2006). *Postpartum Mood and Anxiety Disorders: A Clinician's Guide.* Jones and Bartlett Publishers: Sudbury, MA.

Beck C. T. and Watson S. (2008). Impact of birth trauma on breast-feeding: A tale of two pathways. *Nursing Research* 57, 231.

Bernstein I. H., Rush A. J., Yonkers K., Carmody T. J., Woo A., McConnell K. and Trivedi M. H. (2008). Symptom features of postpartum depression: Are they distinct? *Depression and Anxiety* 25, 20–26.

Colaizzi P. F. (1973). *Reflection and Research in Psychology: A Phenomenological Study of Learning.* Kendall/Hunt Publishing Company: Dubuque, IA.

Colaizzi P. (1978). Psychological research as the phenomenologist views it. In R. Valle and M. King (eds). *Existential Phenomenological Alternative for Psychology.* Oxford University Press: New York, 48–71.

Craig M. and Howard L. M. (2009). Postnatal depression. *Clinical Evidence.* [Online]. Available at: http://www.ncbi.nlm.nih.gov/pmc/articles/PMC2907780/?tool=3 Dpmcentrez=23top= [Accessed 22 April 2011].

Declercq E. R., Sakala C., Corry M. P. and Applebaum S. (2008). *New Mothers Speak Out: National Survey Results Highlight Women's Postpartum Experiences*. Childbirth Connection: New York.

Gavin N., Gaynes B. N., Lohr K .N., Meltzer-Brody S., Gartlehner G. and Swinson T. (2005). Perinatal depression: A systematic review of prevalence and incidence. *Obstetrics and Gynecology* 106, 1071–1083.

Halbreich V. (2005). Postpartum disorders: Multiple underlying mechanisms and risk factors. *Journal of Affective Disorders* 88, 1–7.

Husserl E. (1913). *Ideas Pertaining to a Pure Phenomenology and to a Phenomenological Philosophy: General Introduction to a Pure Phenomenology*. Martinus Nijhoff: The Hague.

Husserl, E. (1960). *Cartesian Meditations* (D. Cairns, trans.). Martinus Nijhoff: The Hague.

Matthey S., Barnett B., Howie P. and Kavanagh D. J. (2003). Diagnosing postpartum depression in mothers and fathers: Whatever happened to anxiety? *Journal of Affective Disorders* 74, 139–147.

Marrs C. R., Durette R. T., Ferraro D. P. and Cross C. L. (2009). Dimensions of postpartum psychiatric distress: Preliminary evidence for broadening clinical scope. *Journal of Affective Disorders* 115, 100–11.

Merleau-Ponty M. (1956). What is phenomenology? *Cross Currents* 6, 59–70.

Reck C., Struben K., Backenstrass M., Stefenelli U., Reinig K., Fuchs T., Sohn C. and Mundt C.(2008). Prevalence, onset and comorbidity of postpartum anxiety and depressive disorders. *Acta Psychiatrica Scandinavica* 118, 459–468.

Ross L. E. and McLean L. M. (2006). Anxiety disorders during pregnancy and the postpartum revealed: A systematic review. *Journal of Clinical Psychiatry* 67, 1285–1298.

Sharma V. (2002). Pharmacotherapy of postpartum depression. *Expert Opinion in Pharmacotherapy* 3, 1421–1431.

Sharma V., Khan M., Corpse C. and Shamra P. (2008). Missed bipolarity and psychiatric comorbidity in women with postpartum depression. *Bipolar Disorders* 10, 742–747.

Spiegelberg H. (1975). *Doing Phenomenology: Essays on and in Phenomenology*. Marinus Nijhoff: The Hague.

12 Heidegger's contribution to hermeneutic phenomenological research

Maria Healy

Introduction

To be known as one of the greatest philosophers of the twentieth century is an immense achievement. Martin Heidegger has been accredited with this accolade by scholars such as Charles Guignon (1993), Richard Palmer (1969), Mark Wrathall (2005) and David Krell (1993). Mark Wrathall (2005) quotes:

> Heidegger did more than any other thinker of the twentieth century to develop a coherent way of thinking and talking about human existence without reducing it to a natural scientific phenomenon or treating it as a ghostly mind haunting the physical world.
>
> (pp. 5–6)

His philosophy has influenced other key intellectuals, including Gadamer, Derrida, Foucault, Sartre and Bourdieu (Guignon 1993). Heidegger's work demonstrates a unique way of understanding the meaning of being in the world (i.e. ontology), that is, human lived experience. This is manifest particularly within his most renowned publication *Being and Time* (*Sein und Zeit*), first published in 1927. Understanding Heidegger's philosophy is central to undertaking Heideggerian hermeneutic phenomenological research. It is therefore important that researchers who claim to be using this approach demonstrate their insight and knowledge of the philosophical underpinnings of Martin Heidegger's work for their research to be substantive and convincing. Indeed, it is argued that only through rigorous interpretive enquiry can valuable meaning be gleaned from the lived experience (Kavanagh 2002).

This chapter seeks to explore and explicate Heidegger's philosophy, beginning with a detailed explanation of its origins and a demonstration of what it is that Heidegger offers to hermeneutic phenomenology. It will examine methods that can be utilized in Heideggerian hermeneutic phenomenological research, giving examples from research which explores Irish women's experiences of postnatal care. Finally, this chapter will discuss briefly how Heidegger's existential concepts can be used to understand and explain phenomena which have come to light during my research. To begin with, a brief chronicle of the life events of Martin Heidegger is offered to place his work and philosophy in context.

Martin Heidegger was born in Messkirch, Germany on 26 September 1889, and he died on 26 May 1976. His father was a manufacturer of barrels and he was also a sexton for the local church. Heidegger went to school initially in Constance (1903–1906) and then in Freiburg from 1906–1909. Here, at the age of 17 he was first introduced to Franz von Brentano's work *On the Manifold Meaning of Being according to Aristotle* (1862) by a pastor from Trinity Church in Constance (Krell 1993). This book stimulated Heidegger's interest into the question of being (Moran and Mooney 2002), and a year later he went on to critically appraise Aristotle's own work, endeavouring to re-read the history of philosophy (Krell 1993). Following a brief period as a Jesuit novitiate, Heidegger enrolled at the University of Freiburg as a theology student and seminarian from 1909–1911. He studied mathematics and then philosophy at Freiburg and it was here that he first encountered the work of Edmund Husserl. Husserl's famous text *Logical Investigations* left a profound impression on Heidegger, yet instilled an inquisitive sense of incorrectness (Moran and Mooney 2002). According to Moran and Mooney (2002) it was around this same period that Heidegger became familiar with hermeneutics through the writings of Schleiermacher, while also engaging with the work of Hölderlin, Rilke, Kierkegaard and Nietzsche. In 1915 Heidegger became a lecturer at Freiburg, was conscripted into the military service from 1915–1918 and later worked as an assistant to Edmund Husserl from 1919–1923. It was in 1923 that he secured the reputation as a great lecturer (as an assistant professor) at Marburg University and afterwards he obtained the appointment to the chair of philosophy at the University of Freiburg in 1928 (Wrathall 2005). For ten months from May 1933 Heidegger joined the Nazi Party. Around the same time he became Rector of Freiburg University until 1934 when he resigned (Krell 1993). After the Second World War, the French military authorities involved in the Allied De-Nazification Committee and faculty from Freiburg University placed Martin Heidegger under rigorous scrutiny due to his involvement with the Nazi party. No firm conclusions were reached by the investigation as to his actual involvement. However, the committee placed a strict ban on Heidegger's freedom to lecture, publish and attend conferences. He found this very difficult and only continued to teach his philosophy in private seminars, with the ban being lifted in 1951, one year before his retirement (Krell 1993, Moran and Mooney 2002). Since then Heidegger's work has been translated into many languages and has gained considerable international recognition. In relation to the significance of Martin Heidegger's philosophy, Mark Wrathall (2005) writes: 'it is not his misadventures with Nazism or his self-importance that is paramount in interpreting his philosophy, but his originality as a thinker and the scope and profundity of his thought itself' (pp. 1–2).

The evolution of Heideggerian hermeneutics

As mentioned above, Heidegger re-read the history of philosophy back to Plato's student, Aristotle (384–322 BC). His intensive study originated from his disagreement with how knowledge had been generated by the philosophical tradition. Aristotle had provided a unique analysis of the question of what 'being' means from an aetiological perspective, believing that there was a unity, as Hanley (2000) describes, 'between what is the case in the world, and what humans correctly perceive to be the case' (p. 203). Signifying logic, Aristotle argued that perception is always interpreted and connected to our experience in the world. This differed from Plato's rationalist belief in disconnected knowledge, which surmized that experience is not required to reveal the truth of an idea (Stevenson 2005). In exploring his theory of perception Aristotle focused on the complex Greek term 'ousía'. Aristotle believed that the 'primary form of being to be investigated is ousía; and ousía is, in the most primary sense, form' (Hanley 2000, p. 67). Thus, the mind thinks about external things: for example, an object is perceived in terms of its form with a shape, the material that it consists of and how the object functions. Aristotle's views were grounded by a belief in God; this led to his argument that there was a certain order or structure in the world and that human beings also have a universal description, or understanding of unity of the ways of being. Heidegger creatively interpreted Aristotle's work (Krell 1993); he disagreed with Aristotle's restricted thinking associated with the categorization of being; in particular the suppressive viewpoint on the individuality of human beings. As Heidegger wrote in *Being and Time,* '...even Aristotle failed to clear away the darkness of these categorical interconnections' (1962, p. 22). The important aspect for Heidegger was not what the unity of these ways of being is, but what 'ousía' (or form) as Aristotle's analogy for the unity of all ways of being actually means (Hanley 2000).

Apart from Heidegger's critical analyses of traditional ontology (the historical philosophical views of being) he also examined in detail Immanuel Kant's (1724–1804) work on transcendental philosophy. Kant believed that space and time and everything associated with these concepts are simply appearances from our world of experience and therefore by discovering the structure and rules of appearance we know the structure of nature itself. Blattner (2006) suggests that Heidegger's adoption of Kant's transcendental turn to ontology transformed his study into the structure and rules of our understanding of being. Subsequently, Heidegger's aim in *Being and Time* was to develop a general ontology of all forms of being by explicating how it is that we understand being.

Historically, Aristotle's philosophy was respected for hundreds of years, until it was dismissed by the Scientific Revolution (Blattner 2006). This change came about by leading philosophers such as Francis Bacon (1561–1626) who had given credence to science as a systematic approach to

discovering knowledge. Heidegger however took issue with the philosophical schools of idealism (where ideas can exist outside the mind) and realism
(where ideas about reality exist in reality outside the mind) and in *Being and
Time* he rejected the entire debate, stating that:

> ...as long as Dasein is (that is, only as long as an understanding of being
> is ontically possible), 'is there' being. When Dasein does not exist [the
> proposition of independent things] can neither be understood nor not
> understood. In such a case even entities within-the-world can neither
> be uncovered nor lie hidden.
>
> (Heidegger 1962, p. 255)

Heidegger also refers to Rene Descartes' (1591–1650) work in *Being and
Time*. Descartes was an influential philosopher of the Renaissance who
through his expertise in mathematical physics provided explanations for a
number of natural occurrences, such as how the heart pumps blood, how
light rays enter the eye into the optical nerve, and so on. Heidegger actually praises Descartes on this aspect of his work as a founder of human
epistemology. Nevertheless, Heidegger comments on Descartes' renowned
stance on dualism:

> Within certain limits the analysis of the extensio [the objective world]
> remains independent of his neglecting to provide an explicit interpre-
> tation for the being of extended entities.
>
> (Heidegger 1962, p. 134)

It is Descartes' belief in dualism that Heidegger rejects outright. The foundation of this is the clear separation between the physical and the metaphysical.
Descartes believes that in order to understand ourselves or to understand
what the 'I' is, we need to extract it from its surroundings so that we can
better comprehend the self for what it is. He stresses in the *Meditations on
First Philosophy* that '...the mind of man is really distinct from the body...'
(Descartes 1979, p. 22). In addition, he goes further to suggest that the body
needs to be separated from the imagination as the sense organs are so close
to the imagination that they can create false perceptions (Descartes 1979).

The genesis of Heidegger's *Being and Time*

Heidegger's indebtedness to the forerunners of phenomenology includes
Frank von Brentano and Edmund Husserl. Heidegger's appreciation is
shown to Husserl by his dedication of *Being and Time* to him and in the foot-
note where he gives recognition to Husserl stating that '...he has also given
us the necessary tools' (Heidegger 1962, p. 490). Frank Brentano, Husserl's
professor had obvious influence on the development of Husserl's phenomenology. Brentano's series of lectures entitled 'Descriptive Psychology' (also

entitled 'Phenomenology') laid emphasis on the accuracy of describing mental states over casual explanations. He claimed that all mental phenomena can be divided into psychical and physical phenomena (Brentano 1995), a view that Husserl rejected (Husserl 1970). Brentano also believed that mental phenomenon can be intentional; that is, they relate to an object whether or not the object thought about really exists (Moran and Mooney 2002). Blattner (2006) further explains that intentionality is 'the mind's capacity to represent the world around it' (p. 2). For example, one might experience being frightened and relate being afraid to some particular thing even if it does not exist. It was the concept of intentionality that Husserl took hold of and developed into his new approach to analysing the experiences of thought and knowing through phenomenology.

In *Logical Investigations,* Husserl identified the necessity to go back to the 'things themselves', to the actual experiences which must have originated in intuition in an effort to understand concepts or ideas of logic (Husserl 1970) (also discussed in Chapters 1 and 4). In developing his philosophy Husserl identified that Brentano may have slipped into assuming that all objects of thought are real, as Blattner (2006) clarifies: 'Once we begin talking about "immanent objects",... it is easy to slide into thinking about meaning as a special sort of thing...' (p. 26). In order to avoid this, Husserl introduced his technique of 'phenomenological reduction' which somehow permits a person to have a change in attitude and suspend their beliefs and assumptions by 'bracketing' them. Husserl uses the Greek term 'epoché' to refer to this period of suspension into the natural attitude. He highlights that this enables pure phenomenology to be undertaken through uninterrupted reflection on experience (Husserl 1981). He states himself this approach can be followed 'by modifying Descartes's method' (Husserl 1981, p. 15); which inevitably gave fuel for Husserl's critics.

According to Theodore Kisiel's (1993) article entitled 'The Genesis of Heidegger's Being and Time' it was Heidegger's move to radically transform Edmund Husserl's work which was the beginning of a more fundamental conception of phenomenology. Martin Heidegger offered a novel way of seeing experience. He critiqued Husserl's philosophy which had followed the traditional stance and in particular rejected his notion of the 'un-living of experience' (Kisiel 1993) that is, bracketing. Instead, he embraced the embedded in the world experience. Kisiel agrees that all that is left after Husserl's objectified methodology is the 'impoverished I-relatedness reduced to a minimum of experiencing' (p. 46).

What is it that Heidegger offers to hermeneutic phenomenology?

Martin Heidegger commenced his work by presenting an ontological analysis of Dasein (which essentially means 'us, human beings') as a way of interpreting the meaning of being and also providing an analysis for the structures of existence. Heidegger notes the task of ontology is to 'explain Being itself and to make the Being of entities stand out in full relief' (Heidegger 1962, p. 49). Thereby Heidegger's methodology pertains only 'To the things themselves!' (p. 50) as experienced by us. He does not accept that his methodology will accidentally stumble on findings. Instead his aim is to uncover existing phenomena, which indicates 'the totality of what lies in the light of day or can be brought to light' (p. 51). In defining logos, the second component of phenomenology, Heidegger indicates that it refers to the making manifest or making sense of what is seen. Thomas Sheehan comments in a podcast interview from KZSU FM radio station Stanford (KZSU 2010) with Robert Harrison entitled 'Heidegger's Being and Time' that Heidegger himself had stressed to him during a meeting in 1971, that:

> Phenomenology is not about things out there ... [it] is about the meaning of things in our world of use, of practical orientation, the significance of things. It is precisely meaning that changes things out there into phenomenon; that is things that meaningful appear to us and that we can engage with.
> (KZSU Stanford 2010, Thomas Sheehan on Heidegger, spoken, 1971)

Heidegger reaffirms that what is understood through his methodology is not the meaning but the entity or the being. Understanding or non-understanding can only take place through Dasein's intelligibility which is structured via the hermeneutic circle (Heidegger 1962). Thus Palmer (1969) asserts that Heidegger's project in *Being and Time* was to deepen and radicalize phenomenology and to explicitly unite it with hermeneutics.[1] Hence Sheehan also comments in the interview with Robert Harrison that it is Dasein who is the hermeneutist, the one who makes sense, and this is a basic characteristic of human beings.

At the beginning of *Being and Time* Heidegger emphasizes that the fundamental nature of Dasein is its existence, and to each one of us our existence is our own. As Heidegger states '...Being, is in each case mine' (Heidegger 1962, p. 67). Heidegger does not mean that Dasein lives in isolation but that Dasein's behaviour potentially demonstrates different modes of being. Thereby 'Dasein is in each case essentially is its own possibility' (p. 68). This includes choice, such as acting authentically or inauthentically.

In division I of *Being and Time* Heidegger explores the world in terms of the entities or substances within it and the way Dasein relates to them. He notes that we have a fundamental perspective on the way we view and understand these entities through our experiences and dealings in our world. He defines them in relation to the way of being which refers to how Dasein makes these entities or substances intelligible. These include: present-at-hand; ready-to-hand; and unready-to-hand. Present-at-hand is everything that is independent of our lives (Blattner 2006), for example substances which are self-sufficient such as trees, an electrical charge or the sun. Ready-to-hand refers to how we do not look at objects as being unrelated to our practical activities but as instrumental objects, such as equipment. Heidegger states:

> The less we just stare at the hammer-thing, and the more we seize hold of it and use it, the more primordial does our relationship to it become, and the more unveiledly is it encountered as that which it is – as equipment.

(Heidegger 1962, p. 98)

Unready-to-hand, Blattner (2006) describes is the 'unavailability of something for use in human practice' (p. 65). When unready-to-hand refers to equipment, there is breakdown or malfunction and we are forced to concentrate on it. Heidegger (1962) stresses that unready-to-hand does not solely pertain to something that is missing or unusable but also relates to that which concerns us greatly and requires our attention.

Heidegger also underlines the importance of incorporating the 'temporal' aspect of being in any attempt to give meaning to the modes and characteristics of being. Understanding entities can therefore only be undertaken in terms of their relation to time of which there are three different modes: the past, present and future (Heidegger 1962). Later in division II of *Being and Time* Heidegger integrates the temporal features that structure Dasein (Blattner 2006).

Dreyfus (1991) summarizes Heidegger's purpose in asking the question of being and highlights that he sought to comprehend our understanding of our practices, by presenting thematically what human beings obliviously do all the time. This is because for Heidegger, a fundamental feature of Dasein's experience is our familiarity with the world that we live in and often do not notice. According to Dreyfus (1991), this was what the philosophical tradition forgot about for over 2000 years. It is central to Heidegger's philosophy. Our familiarity or, in other words, our background is often concealed from us as we frequently take it for granted or become absorbed in our everyday life. Heidegger gives the example of the latch on the door. As we open the door to go out we often do not notice it. Heidegger identified two levels of uncovering a phenomenon: 'ontically' meaning that which is observed and 'ontologically' referring to the phenomenological analysis of the deep structures that underlie and explain the ontic (Frede 1993). He reflects that 'Dasein is ontically "closest" to itself and ontologically farthest; but pre-ontologically it is surely not a stranger' (Heidegger 1962, p. 37). The phrase '…pre-ontologically it is surely not a stranger' is referring to our inability to define our own state of being as we are always currently living in our everyday mode of being, not stopping to analyse it. Consequently, as Sheehan emphasizes, it is only through undertaking fundamental ontology as phenomenology that the question of being can be answered by bringing to light the things that meaningfully appear or are significant to us (KZSU

Stanford 2010). As Heidegger (1962) confirms '...it is itself the clearing' (p. 171), the space left behind after the trees have been cleared away, which illuminates the phenomenon.

As referred to above, Heidegger's philosophy places Dasein (us) as a Being-in-the-world. Using a tripartite formation he identifies three structural elements of being-in-the-world: these include thrownness (facticity); discursiveness; and understanding (projectedness). Thrownness is a basic characteristic of Dasein and refers to the certainty that we as beings find ourselves thrown into a context without having a choice, which is culturally and historically significant (also discussed by Thomson, Chapter 8). Heidegger asserts that the term '..."thrownness" is meant to suggest the facticity of its being delivered over' (p. 174). These somewhat confusing terms refer not just to how the world we live in has an impact on us, but also how we as human beings encounter our world by always being attuned to it and making sense of what matters to us. Blattner (2006) explains that in our being we are '...tuned into the way things matter, our tuning or temper is our mood' (p. 79). Heidegger contends that we are always 'disposed' in a mood (Heidegger 1962).

Discursiveness refers to our activities and how we articulate the world through our language by following the guidelines of interpretation (Guignon 1993). Projectedness refers to our act of understanding, to reach ahead into the meaning of something in order to comprehend it. As humans we cannot take in things and understand them immediately, we have to identify and work things out in terms of something else. For example, a suitcase has the role as a container and transporter for clothes or similar items but is unsuitable to carry liquids. Meaning is therefore only obtained in the projection of which something becomes intelligible as something (Heidegger 1962). Heidegger stresses that '...when something within-the-world is encountered as such, the thing in question already has an involvement which is disclosed in our understanding of the world, and this involvement is one which gets laid out by the interpretation' (p. 190). It is Heidegger's recognition of this background involvement that is unique in comparison to previous traditional philosophers.

Our making sense of things can nevertheless be undertaken in a fallen mode. 'Falling' according to Heidegger (1962) is related to our every day 'absorption in' our activities of life where we don't become fully engaged with our particular responsibilities. The term 'absorption in' reflects our, 'Being-lost in the publicness of the "they" and in this situation we have declined our potential to be authentic and have fallen into the world' (Heidegger 1962, p. 220). Heidegger comments that being 'fallen into the world' is a state in which we act in a programmed way with each other by conforming and not trying to obtain a unique perspective. This is disclosed by three components: idle talk; curiosity; and ambiguity of which every Dasein has the tendency to adhere to. Heidegger believes that when one is 'absorbed in' the 'they' and in the 'world' then one flees from facing up to his or her capability to be authentic. Falling is a situation which most of us can drift into. It is only through uncovering the situation in which we flee that we begin to understand and interpret our being-in-the-world (Heidegger 1962).

The method of Heideggerian hermeneutical phenomenology

The process of Heideggerian hermeneutics as a method of enquiry is circular, as it adheres to the basic principle of the hermeneutical circle which highlights the relatedness of the phenomena under investigation to its surroundings. As described by Palmer (1969) 'The part is understood from the whole and the whole from the inner harmony of its parts' (p. 77). Schleiermacher (1998) who properly credits Friedrich Ast (1778–1841) with asserting the principle '…that everything individual can only be understood via the whole' (p. 70). Heidegger adopted the hermeneutic circle to make interpretation possible, and, in doing so, developed a three-fold structure he called 'the fore-structure of interpretation': 'fore-having, fore-sight and fore-conception'. 'Fore-having', according to Heidegger (1962), is where in every case the interpretation is based on 'something we have in advance' (p. 191), the background context in 'which Dasein knows its way about… in its public environment' (p. 405). For example a new mother may already know from her background knowledge that a baby needs to be fed to survive. 'Fore-sight' refers to the fact that we always enter a situation or experience with a particular view or perspective. 'Fore-conception' is the anticipated sense of the interpretation which becomes conceptualized. For example, when a mother senses that her baby is unwell and later her interpretation is conceptualized when the baby has developed pyrexia. What is most important as emphasized by Heidegger is the 'working out of these fore-structures in terms of the things themselves' (p. 195) so that rigorous interpretation can be possible. It 'is not to get out of the circle [of understanding] but to come into it in the right way' which is essential (p. 195). The process is also reflexive in that the researcher turns a critical gaze towards themselves and how they may have impacted on the research (Finlay 2003). Furthermore, the interpretive process is never ending as it is always tentative, following the assumption that no single correct interpretation exists. Nevertheless the researcher must continually examine the whole and parts of the transcript while frequently listening to the data (if it is in audio format) and with reference to the participants to ensure that the interpretations are reflected in the findings (Diekelmann 2001).

Brief outline of my study

The central aim of my research is to bring to light women's experiences of postnatal care in Ireland. Unlike in Northern Ireland or the United Kingdom, there is no national community midwifery service in the Republic of Ireland. In the study, Heideggerian hermeneutic phenomenology is used to gain a greater understanding of how women experience care following childbirth and give meaning to their experiences. Both primigravid and multigravid women were included, and their postnatal care aspirations and experiences were explored, from the context of inside the hospital and in the community. The research involved two phases (Table 12.1). Phase one consisted of recruiting a cohort of six primigravid women and six multigravid women to participate in three follow-up group interviews. Phase two included a separate cohort of primigravid and multigravid women who participated in individual in-depth interviews. Both research phases followed a longitudinal approach to data collection. The stages were from 28 to 38 weeks antenatally, and from two to eight weeks and three to four months postpartum. The collection of data and the interpretive method involved a number of processes, which are outlined below.

The hermeneutic group interview

Group interviews provide 'neutral controls on data collection' as participants challenge or question extreme viewpoints (Robinson 1999), validate information given by others, and allow the moderator to probe for deeper levels of information (Lane *et al.* 2001). Group interviews were chosen as the initial method of data collection to scope the research field and identify care issues concerning the women that may need further in-depth enquiry in phase two, while ensuring that the phenomenological conversations were not inhibited. As described by Smythe *et al.* (2008) 'Our interviewing style is not structured in that we follow a pre-organised plan, nor unstructured, where we go with no clear sense of why we are there...but always an interview is about something' (p. 1392). This data collection strategy promoted an in-depth, interpretative dialogue as encouraged by Benner (1994) who emphasizes that data collection, enquiry, and analysis should not be separated.

Table 12.1 Number of participants involved at the different stages and phases of data collection

Stages of data collection	Phase one: No. of participants in primigravid group interview	Phase one: No. of participants in multiparous group interview	Phase two: No. of participants in primigravid individual interviews	Phase two: No. of participants in multiparous individual interviews
28 to 38 weeks antenatally	6	6	7	6
2 to 8 weeks postnatally	5	4	5	5
3 to 4 months postnatally	5	4	5	5
Total	6 group interviews		33 individual interviews	

Indeed the actual group interview process encouraged a dynamic that triggered the sharing of postnatal care experiences through recollection and self-reflection, when otherwise the participants may have remained silent. A sense of solidarity also prevailed, and, in some cases, the group process appeared to have a therapeutic effect for some participants, particularly when there was an acknowledgement of similar experiences.

Benner (1994) emphasizes the effectiveness of using the small group interview in a hermeneutic phenomenological study of health and illness, stating that group interviews can achieve several purposes such as:

- creating a natural communicative context for telling stories from practice
- providing a rich basis for active listening
- meanings of the participants' stories can be enriched by stories triggered to counter, contrast, or bring up similarities
- simulating a work environment that creates a forum for thinking and talking about work situations.

The hermeneutic individual interview

Highlighting the purpose of the phenomenological interview, Sorrell Dinkins (2005) states the aim is to 'understand a phenomenon by drawing from the respondent(s) a vivid picture of the "lived experience", complete with the richness of detail and context that shape the experience' (p. 113). The communicative context therefore must prevent the participants from feeling awkward or constrained by the interview process, particularly by the use of foreign or abstract language (Benner 1994). In order to achieve this, 2 to 3 days prior to both the group and the individual interviews taking place I contacted the participants to remind them of the interview and to encourage them to recollect their postnatal care experiences prior to our meeting. This proved fruitful in the richness of the transcripts. The majority of the interviews were held at the participants' home. At the beginning of each interview the participants were asked a broad open hermeneutical question to elicit their postnatal care story and to seek their interpretation(s) on the meanings and significances of their experience: 'Can you please tell me about your postnatal care experience(s) and what does it mean to you to have had this experience?' Once their story was recounted, open prompt questions were used to clarify words or phrases used by the participants that had taken for granted meaning, for example: 'care' or 'support'. In addition, to avoid causal relationships and explanations the participants were asked to give an example(s) of their experience(s). Another approach used to seek the meanings and significances of the women's postnatal care experience(s) was to ask them: 'If they had a close relative who would soon be in a similar situation to themselves, having just had a baby what would they say to them about postnatal care?' These detailed descriptions of the practices and shared meanings are according to Diekelmann and Ironside (1998) '...intended to reveal, enhance, or extend understandings of the human situation as it is lived' (p. 343).

To further ensure that a comprehensive approach to the hermeneutic interviewing was undertaken the 'Socratic-Hermeneutic Inter-view' as described by Sorrell Dinkins (2005) was followed when appropriate. This alternative approach to phenomenological interviews incorporates Socrates' ideas of shared inquiry were the focus is moved away from the 'respondent' to '...a shared dialogue focused on reflections of both interviewer and the interviewee as they share ideas, listen, and reflect together, thus forming an inter-view' (p. 128). This approach was applicable particularly when I, the interviewer, was in the postnatal period myself having recently given birth. Principally, each interview was unique and, what was most important, had '...openness to what "is" – to the play of conversation' (Smythe *et al.* 2008, p. 1392).

Data analysis

Prior to data analysis, each interview was transcribed verbatim by the same audio typist and checked for accuracy against the audio by myself. Each interview was read in its entirety. As the process of hermeneutic phenomenological analysis is iterative and non-linear, broad, sweeping themes were initially identified across interviews with the aid of MAXQDA2, a computer software package for data management. The specific analytical approach used for both the group interviews and the individual interviews followed the methods proposed by Crist and Tanner (2003). They highlight a number of phases that can be followed to assist in approaching this interpretive process as systematically as possible, although the authors stress that the phases may overlap. These include:

Phase 1: Early focus and lines of enquiry

This includes a critical evaluation of the researcher's interview and field notes within the transcripts. Lines of enquiry from initial interpretations guide subsequent interviews and direct future sampling to provide deeper, richer understanding.

Phase 2: Central concerns, exemplars and paradigm cases

The interpretive researcher or team identify central concerns, important themes, or meanings, that are unfolding for specific informants. This process begins with interpretive writing of approximately three to five page summaries of central concerns with salient excerpts. A review of new or revised summaries may cause exemplars and paradigm cases to emerge. Exemplars are excerpts that define common themes or meaning across informants, whereas paradigm cases are vibrant stories or strong instances of particular patterns of meaning.

Phase 3: Shared meanings

As informants' central concerns become clear, the researcher/team members observe shared meanings within and across stories.

Phase 4: Final interpretations

Subsequent interpretive notes and summaries continue to provide a line of enquiry for current narratives and future sampling. In-depth interpretations are developed and final interviews address pending lines of enquiry.

Phase 5: Dissemination of the interpretation

This phase continues to follow an iterative process between the narrative, field notes and input from the researcher/team, as interpretations are refined for publication.

During each of these phases time was taken to identify the interpretative decisions and recommendations. These became part of the research log as an audit trail. It is important that the hermeneutic phenomenologist ensures that he/she does not misinterpret participants' responses. Plager's (1994) principles for evaluating findings from a hermeneutic phenomenological study were adhered to in my study; these include the following.

- Coherence: the account presents a unified picture, including letting contradictions show up and making as much sense of them as the text will allow.
- Comprehensiveness: the account must give a sense of the whole that is the context (situatedness) and temporality for the participants.
- Penetration: the account 'attempts to resolve a central problematic' (p. 29).
- Thoroughness: the account deals with all the questions posed.
- Appropriateness: the questions must be those raised by the text itself.
- Contextuality: the historical and contextual nature of the text must be preserved.
- Agreement: the account must agree with what the text says (not attempt a hermeneutic of suspicion) but should reserve room for reinterpretation by showing where previous interpretations were deficient.
- Suggestiveness: a good understanding in the interpretive account will raise questions to stimulate further interpretive research.

The researcher has a key role as highlighted above, in that he or she writes themselves into the process through reflection on their experience of data collection and analysis. By keeping a study diary as emphasized by (Gadamer 1976), I was able to leave a decision trail on the theoretical, methodological and analytical choices I made throughout the study.

Using Heidegger's existential concepts

Within division I of *Being and Time* Heidegger articulates a phenomenology of everyday life. Later on in division II he presents existential themes that represent an exploration into how we as human beings can change in light of our experience with the extreme challenges of life (Blattner 2006). His philosophy can thereby provide conceptual insights that can be used to understand and explain phenomenon which have come to light during hermeneutic phenomenological research. Three themes from my research into women's experiences of postnatal care in Ireland are presented here to illustrate how Heideggerian concepts can help to illuminate interpretations. These include: 'moods'; 'unready-to-hand'; and 'being-with'. All names used are pseudonyms.

Moods

For Heidegger, moods, or attunement, are a basic characteristic of our familiarity with the world. Heidegger (1962) claims that 'A mood assails us. It comes neither from "outside" nor from "inside" but arises out of Being-in-the world' (p. 176). Moods have an effect on the atmosphere and can be a monitor how we are 'faring', or as Heidegger writes, 'how we are doing' (p. 173). Our moods are also passive to us, as they are often affected by the situation we find ourselves in. Heidegger uses the term 'disposedness' to explain what is common to all moods and how moods for us are related to being-in-the-world. Using fear as an example of a mood Heidegger describes three essential characteristics of disposedness: First, disposedness discloses our thrownness, our inability to control certain circumstances in the world; disposedness also 'discloses being-in-the-world as a whole', as when we are frightened for example certain features of our situation are more dominant than others and finally, a facet of disposedness is our 'submission to the world': that is, when we find ourselves in a vulnerable situation, certain possibilities matter more or are more important to us than others. Moods therefore can import or disclose the way things, persons or events matter to us. This Heideggerian concept became apparent in my interpretations as per the comments from research participants Marie and Claire – it is the little touches that matter to them:

> …particularly for second time mothers, when you don't necessarily need to be shown how to do stuff you just need a little bit of isn't this a wonderful time of your life kind of experience, and here's a cup of tea.
> (Marie)

Oh it's very important to have your name, for me it was really important that my name was being used…in the [postnatal] ward it nearly, it kind of makes me laugh about the Mum thing, you know, you're just Mum up there, you know, there's no name when you're up on the ward, it's like 'Mum do this'.

(Claire)

Unready-to-hand

As mentioned above, Heidegger's concept of unready-to-hand pertains to a breakdown situation or a malfunction which we are forced to concentrate on. It also relates to that which concerns us greatly and requires our attention. For some of the women in my research, becoming a new mother was very challenging, particularly when they felt unprepared. These findings mirror Heidegger's unready-to-hand concept. Below Annie describes the 'horrendous' experience of her first night at home with her new baby:

… our first night home was horrendous because I really didn't know what to expect, because nobody told me what to expect and …, we didn't know what we were doing for changing and I got very frustrated and Michael got very frustrated on that first night because we didn't know how difficult it was going to be. And I suppose [the baby] fed off that a little bit as well and he was probably a bit anxious as well and it was horrendous and I thought, I can't do this, I cannot do this!, this is just, I am too tired!, I am too emotional!, I cannot do this and Michael was the same.

(Annie)

Sarah explains her concern about her husband's inability to bond with their baby who suffers from colic:

Sean just didn't bond with her at all, I think only really in the last two weeks he's started to make some connection with her, he just said she's not like other babies, she doesn't smile, she doesn't look at you. She used to not make eye-contact; she was so distracted with the pain [colic]… Sean just used to say I just want my life back and that used to really hurt me because I'd think oh she'll be better, …and I was trying to make excuses for her saying she'll be better soon, it'll be gone in three months and then when three months came and it didn't go …I mean obviously I found the crying hard, looking at her struggling but I didn't find it hard to make a relationship with her as such, but Sean really did…

(Sarah)

Heidegger emphasizes that 'Anything which is un-ready-to-hand in this way is disturbing to us' (Heidegger 1962, p. 103).

Being-with

The concept of 'being-with' for Heidegger (1962) is a characteristic of each individual Dasein as it is an 'existential constituent of Being-in-the world' (p. 163) that of our being with others. We can still be with others and be alone, as people who are significant to us do not always have to be near. As others matter to us, the concern we have as we comport ourselves towards them Heidegger refers to as 'solicitude' or 'Fürsorge', which is translated as 'caring-for'. This manner of caring-for which Dasein demonstrates in being-with others is completely opposite to the concern or 'Besorge' that ready-to-hand or present-at-hand entities receive as objects of concern. Heidegger writes 'Thus as Being-with, Dasein "is" essentially for-the-sake-of others' (1962, p. 160). He also confirms that 'solicitude proves to be a state of Dasein's Being' (1962, p. 159), particularly as there are different modes of solicitude, ranging from the deficient or indifferent to the positive. According to Heidegger, positive modes of caring for other can be 'inauthentic', defined as a 'leaping in' for the other, a 'taking care' of their possibilities for them rendering them dependent (also refer to Chapter 3). This is opposed to 'authentic' caring, whereby there is a freeing of the other for their own possibilities.

Some of the women in the study experienced authentic care, as described by Jane:

> Well they [the midwife] would make a point of asking me had I had some sleep, had I eaten, how was he [the baby], how was I feeling, you know, all that type of thing and then there was, you know, the physical check up as well, they did all of that and as I say, in that kind of a nice chatty way, it wasn't an interrogation of anything ... you felt like it was more of a friend and a chat and so I think you were more likely to be open with them.
>
> (Jane)

This authentic caring for the new mother helps build maternal agency and exhibits the core element of being a midwife and as per the International Confederation of Midwives definition of a midwife (ICM 2005). Theresa explains below how she responded when a midwife demonstrated an indifferent aspect of solicitude and highlights the subsequent outcome:

> When I knew a midwife wasn't interested I just didn't bother engaging with them, you know, I didn't really ask them anything.
>
> (Theresa)

In summary, by utilizing the Heideggerian existential concepts during the interpretation phase I was able to illuminate how the women's postnatal care was experienced and internalized.

Conclusion

Heidegger's contribution to the genesis and development of hermeneutic phenomenology is momentous. He has provided a philosophy, created the basis for a methodology, outlined the hermeneutical method, and provided existential concepts which can be utilized to understand and explain phenomenon. By fully comprehending the underpinnings of Heidegger's work the hermeneutic phenomenological researcher can uncover insightful meanings and significances of phenomena for those who experience it.

Note

1 The term hermeneutics originates from Greek mythology whereby a great messenger of the gods named Hermes not only communicated verbatim the messages he was given by the gods, but also interpreted their meaning for the people. According to Bleicher (1980), hermeneutics was used from an early stage to assist with understanding the language of a text, to facilitate biblical exegesis, and to guide jurisdiction.

References

Benner P. (1994) *Interpretative Phenomenology: Embodiment, Caring and Ethics in Health and Illness.* Sage Publications: California.

Blattner W. (2006) *Heidegger's Being and Time.* Continuum: London.

Bleicher J. (1980) *Contemporary Hermeneutics: Hermeneutics as Method, Philosophy and Critique.* Routledge & Kegan Paul: London.

Brentano (1995) *Psychology from an Empirical Standpoint* (2nd edn), (trans. Rancurrello A.C., Terrell D.B. and McAlister. L.L.). Routledge: London.

Crist J.D. and Tanner C.A. (2003) Interpretation/analysis methods in hermeneutic interpretive phenomenology. *Nursing Research* 52, 202–205.

Descartes R. (1979) *Mediations on First Philosophy.* Hackett Publishing: Indianapolis.

Diekelmann N.L. (2001) Narrative Pedagogy: Heideggerian Hermeneutical Analyses of Lived Experiences of Students, Teachers, and Clinicians. *Advance Nursing Science* 23, 53–71.

Diekelmann N. and Ironside P. (1998) 'Hermeneutics'. In: *Encyclopaedia of Nursing Research* (ed. J. Fitzpatrick). Springer: New York.

Dreyfus H.L. (1991) *Being-in-the-World: A Commentary on Heidegger's Being and Time, Division I.* The MIT Press: Massachusetts.

Finlay L. (2003) The reflexive journey: mapping multiple routes. In: *Reflexitvity: A Practical Guide for Researchers in Health and Social Sciences.* (eds. L. Finlay and B. Gough), 3–20. Blackwell Publishing: Oxford.

Frede D. (1993) The question of being: Heidegger's project. In: *The Cambridge Companion to Heidegger* (ed. C. Guignon), 42–69. Cambridge University Press: Cambridge.

Gadamer H.G. (1976) *Philosophical Hermeneutics,* (trans. D.E. Linge). University of California: Berkeley.

Guignon C. (ed.) (1993) *The Cambridge Companion to Heidegger.* Cambridge University Press: Cambridge.

Hanley C. (2000) *Being and God in Aristotle and Heidegger: The Role of Method in Thinking the Infinite*. Rowman & Littlefield Publishers, Inc: Lanham.

Heidegger M. (1962) *Being and Time*. (trans. J. Macquarrie and E. Robinson). Harper Collins: New York (original work published 1927).

Husserl E. (1970) *Logical Investigations* (trans. J.N. Findlay). Routledge: London.

Husserl E. (1981) *Husserl: Shorter Works*, (eds P. Mc Cormick and F. Elliston, trans. R. Welsh Jordan). University of Notre Dame/Harvester Press: Notre Dame.

International Confederation of Midwives (2005) *Definition of the Midwife*. Adopted at the International Confederation of Midwives Council meeting, 19th July, Brisbane, Australia.

Kavanagh K.H. (2002) Foreword In: *First, do no Harm: Power, Oppression and Violence in Healthcare* (ed. N.L. Diekelmann), xiii–xv. The University of Wisconsin Press: Madison.

Kisiel T. (1993) *The Genesis of Heidegger's Being and Time*. University of California Press: Berkeley.

Krell D.F. (1993) *Martin Heidegger: Basic Writings*, Harper San Francisco: New York.

KZSU Stanford (2010) Entitled opinions – about life and literature: *Heidegger's Being and Time* Thomas Sheehan interviewed by. [Online]. Tuesday 18 May. Available at: http://french-italian.stanford.edu/opinions/ [Accessed 21 May 2010].

Lane P., McKenna H., Ryan A. and Fleming P. (2001) Focus group methodology. *Nurse Researcher* 8(3): 45–59.

Moran D. and Mooney T. (2002) (eds) *The Phenomenology Reader*, Routledge: London.

Palmer R. (1969) *Hermeneutics: Interpretation Theory in Schleiermacher, Dilthey, Heidegger, and Gadamer*. Northwestern University Press: Evanston.

Plager K.A. (1994) Hermeneutic phenomenology: a methodology for family health and health promotion study in nursing. In Benner P. (ed.) *Interpretative Phenomenology: embodiment, caring and ethics in health and illness*. Sage: Thousand Oaks, California.

Robinson L. (1999) The use of focus groups methodology with selected examples from sexual health research. *Journal of Advanced Nursing* 29, 905–913.

Schleiermacher F. (1998) *Hermeneutics and Criticism. Cambridge Texts in the History of Philosophy* (trans. and ed. A. Bowie). Cambridge University Press: Cambridge.

Sorrell Dinkins C.S. (2005) Shared inquiry Socratic-Hermeneutic Interpre-viewing. In *Beyond Method: Philosophical Conversations in Healthcare Research and Scholarship* (ed. P.M. Ironside), The University of Wisconsin Press: Madison.

Stevenson J. (2005) *The Complete Idiot's Guide to Philosophy*, 3rd edn. Alpha: New York.

Smythe E.A., Ironside P.M., Sims S.L., Swenson M.M. and Spence D.G. (2008) Doing Heideggerian hermeneutic research: A discussion paper. *International Journal of Nursing Studies* 45, 1389–1397.

Wrathall, M. (2005) *How to read Heidegger*. W. W. Norton & Company: New York.

13 Authenticity and poetics

What is different about phenomenology?

Gill Thomson, Fiona Dykes and Soo Downe

I imagine this midnight moment's forest:
Something else is alive
Beside the clock's loneliness
And this blank page where my fingers move ...

... Across clearings, an eye,
A widening deepening greenness,
Brilliantly, concentratedly,
Coming about its own business

Till, with a sudden sharp hot stink of fox
It enters the dark hole of the head.
The window is starless still; the clock ticks,
The page is printed.

(Ted Hughes)

Introduction

In 1998, Geanellos made a plea for those who intend to use phenomenology for research to understand the philosophical underpinning both of the methodology itself, and of the specific phenomenological approach adopted (Geanellos 1998). It seems that the tide has not yet turned in this respect. This is problematic, as there is a risk that 'phenomenology' might become identified with qualitative research in general – 'I'm looking for meaning, so it must be phenomenology'. As Therese Bondas states (refer to Chapter 1): 'phenomenological methods should not be forced to fit circumstances where they are not appropriate'. This being said, once the fundamental principles are adhered to, there is no uniquely correect method that must be adopted in phenomenological research. There are, however, features that could be argued to be the hallmark of genuinely phenomenological studies. In this chapter, two of these are explored: evidence of authenticity, and an attention to poetics. These fundamentals, and some of the concepts associated with them, are threaded through the work of the authors presented here. All the chapters have been independently written and subject to conventional peer review: in this chapter, some of them are brought together to illustrate the nature and importance of these cardinal features.

Authenticity

The intention of this book has been to demonstrate the potential and range of phenomenology as a research method in all its guises. Possibly more importantly, we have aimed to show that phenomenology is, at its root, a philosophy. Indeed, as Maria Healy (Chapter 12) demonstrates in her inter-weaving of Heidegger's biography with the emergence of his philosophy of interpretive phenomenology, it is intrinsically linked to our historicity. Making the decision to adopt a phenomenological perceptive is therefore not merely a methodological choice, but one that carries an implicit set of values. It is not a neutral standpoint. Indeed, taking a phenomenologi-cal route explicitly requires authenticity, and a retreat from 'fallenness'. Researchers who walk hand in hand with phenomenological philosophers cannot just 'do' research; just as Heidegger's philosophical turn does not allow individuals to just 'live' their lives. Instead, this road requires an effort to authentically engage with what could be, rather than simply describing what is. In an extension of this sensibility, Mel Duffy (Chapter 5) uses the term 'bad faith' as coined by Sartre for a kind of inauthenticity that does not choose to recognize and see the Other (in this case lesbian women) as different and of value. For maternity care, the insistence on moving from a 'fallen' state where life is lived routinely and inauthentically/in bad faith is a clarion call to 're-enchantment', in response to Weber's notion of a modernist 'disenchanted world' . For those who follow Husserl and the lifeworld approach, this need for authentic self-reflexivity (or 'bri-dling' as proposed by Karin Dahlberg in Chapter 2) is played out in the requirements for bracketing. This reveals pre-understandings, and forces individuals to surface their views and beliefs, to render them visible, and to face any potentially inauthentic reluctance to deal with them. Therese Bondas illustrates this point, when she records her surprise at finding that some of her respondents viewed their pregnant bodies as disgusting, in contrast to her own sense of the beauty and positive power of pregnancy and birth (Chapter 1).

Alongside this, the concepts of 'massiveness' and 'machination' were originally Heideggerian critiques of industrialization. As Gill Thomson illus-trates in her exploration of the meaning of traumatic birth (Chapter 8), they can serve equally well as a critique of inauthentic reductionism in maternity care – of the distillation of all human experience into one, risk averse way of doing things, and a rejection of creativity, variation, uncertainty, innova-tion, and trial and error. As Gill notes, massiveness 'enframes' experience as something to be standardized, neutralized, controlled and passionless, so that, eventually: 'the frenzied-ness of ordering... blocks...revealing and so radically endangers…. the essence of truth'. Acknowledging this opens the potential to find ways to deal with it. In this respect, a genuine acceptance of the philosophy of phenomenology increases the potential to authentically engage with change in the maternity services, at all levels: to move away from 'semblance' in Elizabeth Smythe's words (Chapter 3). As a consequence, there is a turn away from making excuses for how things are: to stop dis-sembling, and to move genuinely towards the thing itself. In this case, this brings us closer to a genuine understanding of the meaning of childbirth experiences for mother, baby, family and society.

Poetics

The second hallmark, that of poetics, is illustrated in the poem fragment at the beginning of the chapter. In the poem, Ted Hughes is writing about the act of the emergence of the poem itself. As the words track the emergence of a fox from the darkness, the poem is created. The work is both a methodological treatise, and the thing itself – the poem. This is a perfect metaphor for the emergence of the phenomenological insight – the reaching for the essence of Being. The final phenomenological analysis should be the opposite of reductionism. Where this is achieved, the themes that emerge are not just descriptive categories, but concentrated nuggets of meaning that, when read, explode in the brain into nuanced and complex insights into the phenomenon under investigation. As Elizabeth Smythe notes: 'Meaning lies between the lines of what is said, to be uncovered' (Chapter 3). When the phenomena are 'enframed' effectively, they cast a blinding light onto 'the truth' – far from being endangered, it is illuminated, and made possible by being made visible. Examples in this book include Ingela Lundgren's 'releasing and relieving encounters', and 'anchored companion' (Chapter 7); Joyce Cowan's personification of preeclampsia as it hides, announces, and dissembles (Chapter 6); and Gill Thomson's use of the Heideggerian term 'Abandonment of Being' as a catalyst for understanding what women traumatized by childbirth think and feel (Chapter 8). As Lauren Hunter states in Chapter 10:

> Heidegger considered 'language to be the house of our Being'; he perceived that poetry provides not only a source of aesthetic pleasure, but has the power to reveal our world and transform our existence.
>
> (Polt 2003, p. 177)

Conclusion

A decision to use phenomenology is not then, one to be taken lightly. Carried out appropriately, it entails a genuine desire to engage with the Other, and a view of life as a whole, and not just as the fragment of time under scrutiny in a particular research study. Taken in this vein, it becomes something that is potentially life-changing and always, when done skillfully, life-enhancing. The authors in this book have demonstrated how this can be done. It is now over to you, the readers, to take the next step in your own phenomenological encounters. We wish you the very best with your particular endeavors.

> To romanticize the world is to make us aware of the magic, mystery and wonder of the world; it is to educate the senses to see the ordinary as extraordinary, the familiar as strange, the mundane as sacred, the finite as infinite.

> (Novalis, cited in Beiser 1998)

References

Beiser F.C. (1998) 'A Romantic Education: The Concept of Bildung in Early German Romanticism'. In Rorty, A.O. (ed) *Philosophers on Education: Historical Perspectives.* pp. 294. Routledge: London.

Geanellos R. (1998) Hermeneutic philosophy. Part I: Implications of its use as methodology in interpretive nursing research. *Nursing Inquiry* 5 (3), 154–63.

Index

Note: Page numbers followed by 'f' refer to figures and followed by 't' refer to tables.